# THE TRIATHLON
## TRAINING BOOK

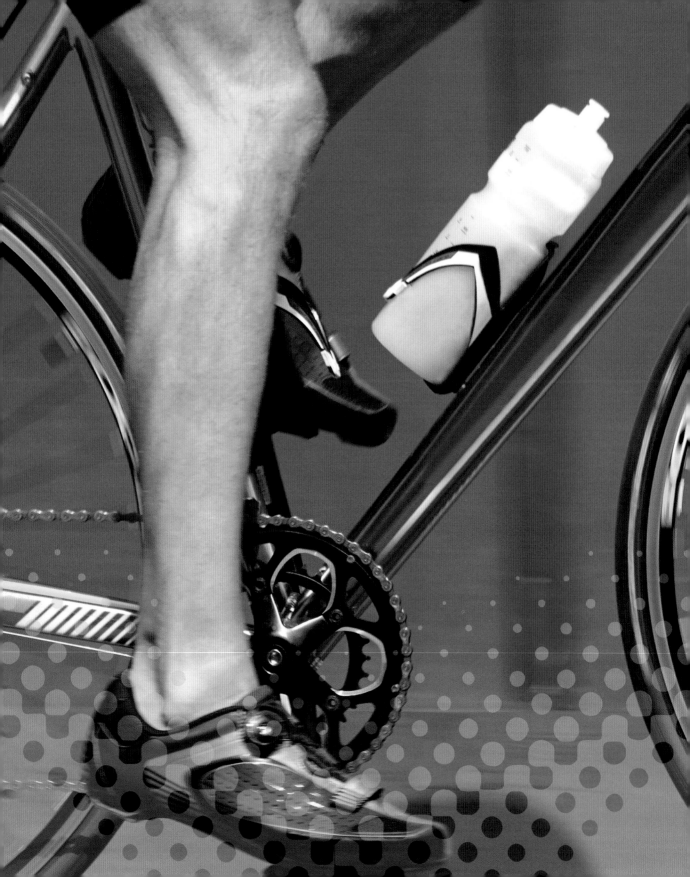

# THE TRIATHLON TRAINING BOOK

James Beckinsale MSc

**Senior Editor**
Camilla Hallinan

**Project Art Editor**
Katherine Raj

**Project Editor**
Martha Burley

**Pre-Production Producer**
Rebecca Fallowfield

**Editors**
Hazel Beynon
Niki Foreman
Liz Jones
Simon Mugford
Steve Setford

**Producer**
Stephanie McConnell

**Jackets Team**
Francesca Young
Harriet Yeomans

**Editorial Assistant**
Alice Kewellhampton

**Creative Technical Support**
Sonia Charbonnier

**Managing Editor**
Stephanie Farrow

**Managing Art Editor**
Christine Keilty

**Produced by** DesignForge.ink

**Photography**
John Davis

**Illustrator**
Phil Gamble

First published in Great Britain in 2016 by
Dorling Kindersley Limited
80 Strand, London WC2R 0RL

ISBN 978-0-2412-2977-4

Printed and bound in China

All images © Dorling Kindersley Limited
For further information see: www.dkimages.com

A WORLD OF IDEAS:
SEE ALL THERE IS TO KNOW

www.dk.com

# CONTENTS

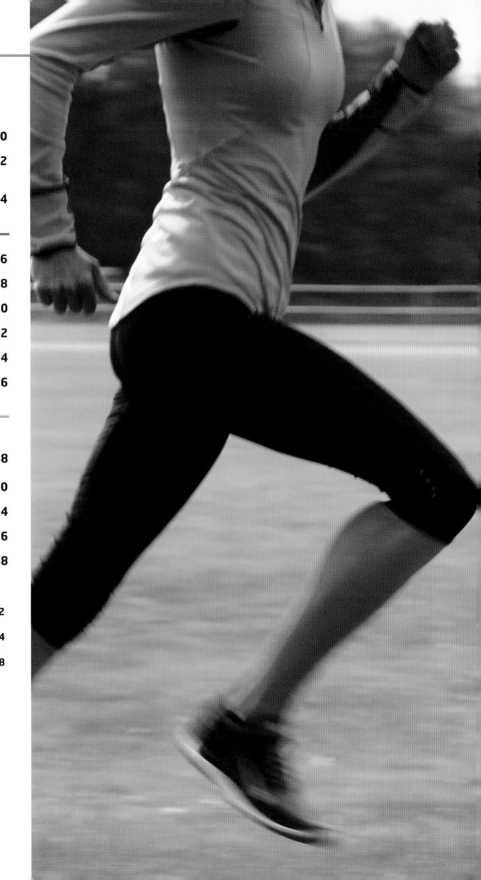

# INTRODUCTION

**Triathlon is now one** of the world's fastest-growing sports. Awareness has grown and grown since its inclusion in the 2000 Sydney Olympics, and there is now television coverage across more than 160 countries. It's hardly surprising that more people than ever are – like you – keen to take part in this fantastic and rewarding sport.

## THE PROFESSIONALS

Watching Olympic-distance triathlon on TV is both exciting and awe-inspiring. There's nothing like the thrill of seeing a group of super-fit endurance athletes dive into a beautiful stretch of ocean, lake, or river for the swim. Soon they are out of the water and running into transition, ripping off wetsuits, caps, and goggles and putting on their helmets. Once they have grabbed their bikes, they perform a "flying mount" and head off to cycle at speeds of close to 40kph (25mph) for women and 45kph (28mph) for men. Finally they come to the last section. Having discarded their bikes and helmets, and pulled on their trainers (all in around 45 seconds flat), they head out of transition at a blistering pace for the run.

The more you learn about triathlon the more you admire these athletes. You'll notice them using all the tactics available to conserve energy, stay out of trouble, and overtake the competition, or realise how fast you have to run to cover 10km in under 35 minutes. It's exhilarating, dynamic, and inspiring.

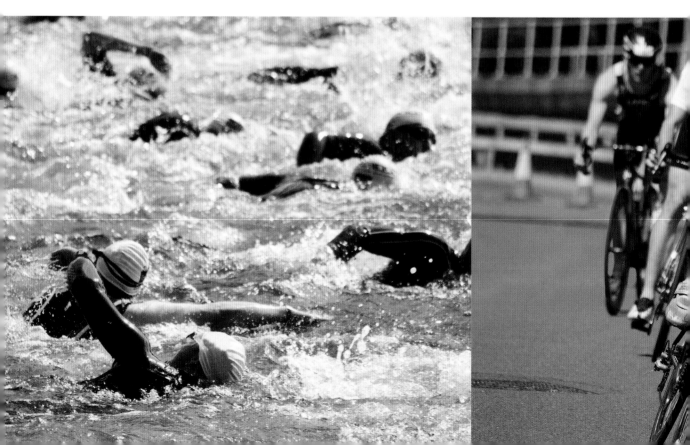

## THE NOVICES

There is, of course, another side to triathlon. It can be just as inspiring to watch novice triathletes swimming breaststroke for 400m in a pool. After the swim leg, they walk to their bikes, perhaps already tired, put their socks on in transition (maybe adding a warmer top), and then walk with their bikes to the mount line for the cycle section. If there's a tailwind, they may be able to complete 20km at a speed of around 20kph (12mph). After the bike section, they return to transition for the last leg, all the time wondering how on earth they will manage a 5km run!

However, somehow they do manage it, because not only is this the grass roots of triathlon, it is an expression of the human spirit and what we can achieve with a little grit and determination.

## A LIFESTYLE CHOICE

There is, of course, also a middle ground between the novice and the elite athlete. Some triathletes dedicate more than 15 hours per week to training, while juggling a full-time job, family commitments, and a social life.

One of the biggest attractions of triathlon is that it can be a great lifestyle sport – you train as much as you can and when you can. You don't need to train as much as the highly dedicated; you can just go to your local pool for a 30-minute swim a couple of times a week, cycle to and from work, and go jogging with your family at weekends or in the evenings. If that is all you can do, that's fine. It will be more than enough training to get you around a sprint-distance triathlon course.

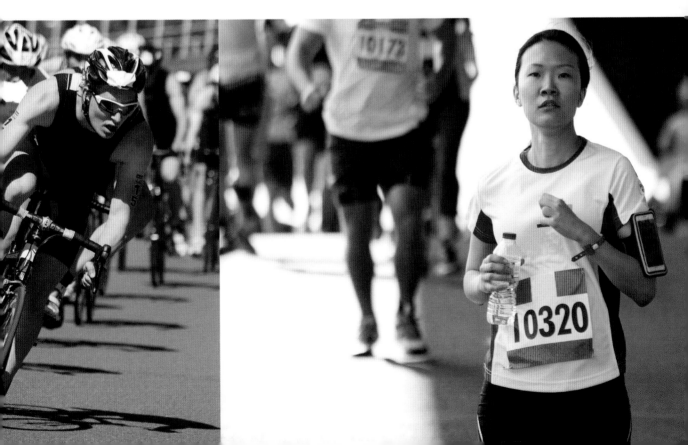

## SOMETHING FOR EVERYONE

There are four main triathlon distances: Sprint, Olympic, Half Ironman, and Ironman. Every athlete, from novice to professional, will have their own particular preference. Different distances require different skill levels, and therefore different levels of training and preparation, but there is something to suit everyone (see pp.124-131).

**The four main triathlon distances:**

**Sprint** (750m swim - 20km bike - 5km run)

**Olympic** (1500m swim - 40km bike - 10km run)

**Half Ironman** or 70.3 (1900m swim - 90km bike - 21km run)

**Ironman** (3.8km swim - 180km bike - 42km run)

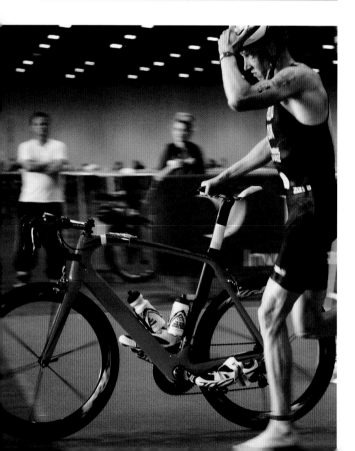

Many athletes come to triathlon from other sports, while some have no sporting background at all. Others are just looking for a new challenge. I was a boxer. When I started triathlon training at 25 I had never cycled competitively and couldn't even swim!

As a coach, I found that my initial lack of experience gave me an edge – I had to master all three disciplines myself before moving into coaching. So I understand what it's like not to "feel the water", or have legs screaming with fatigue from the bike. That said, I would have preferred not to have been the last person out of the water when I competed at the World Triathlon Championships in Canada in 1999,

Despite that, some twenty years later I am still competing in triathlon and coaching full time – and I still believe I have the best job in the world.

As you go through the book, you will learn the intricacies of the swimming, cycling, and running techniques, discovering why - for me at least - each is its own art form. But I have also tried to combine art with science. I'll explain how you can use the training programmes provided to train efficiently - what to eat, what to drink, when to recover, and how to tailor training sessions to fit into your lifestyle. I'll also cover how to avoid common injuries and how to deal with those that occur. Finally, I'll explain how to prepare physically and psychologically for the race itself, so you're at your peak when you need to be.

Whether you have a coach or you're a member of a triathlon club, you'll be able to use the knowledge you gain from this book at every stage of your training, learning and building confidence as you improve. I am still learning new things and love the challenges that this fantastic sport brings me every day. I hope you will too.

Let's get training!

**James Beckinsale**
MSc, BTA L3

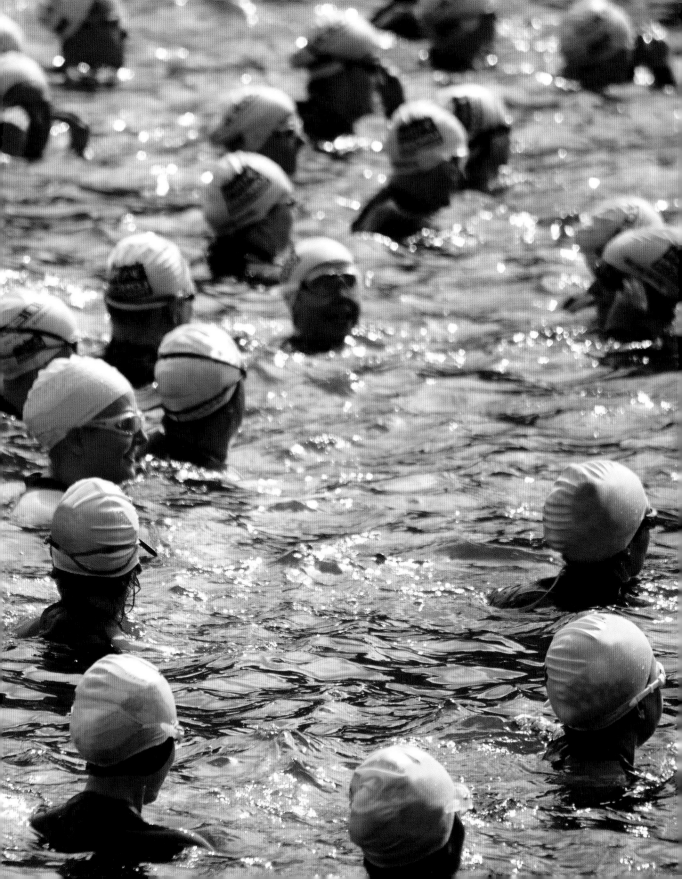

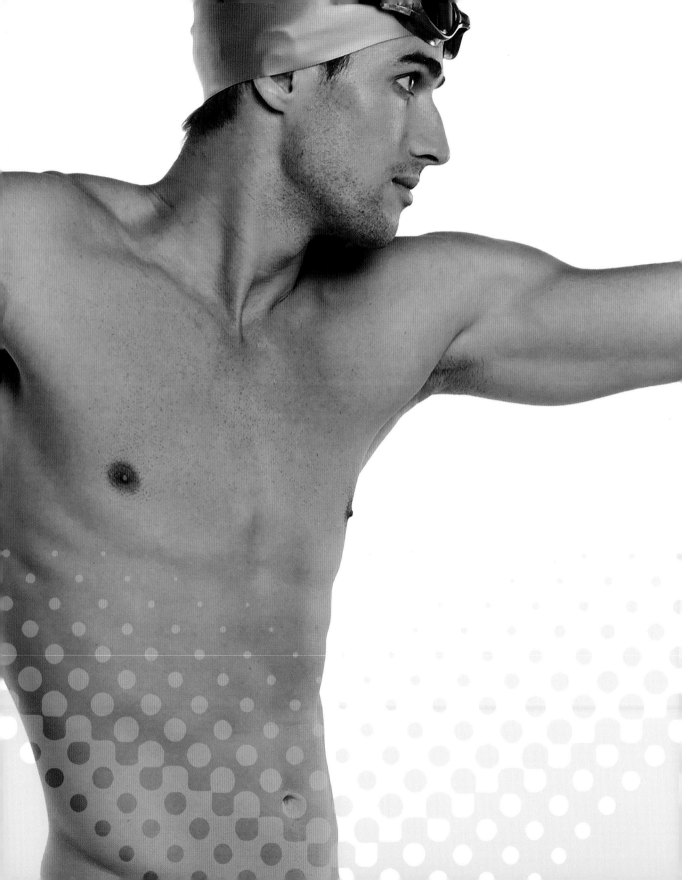

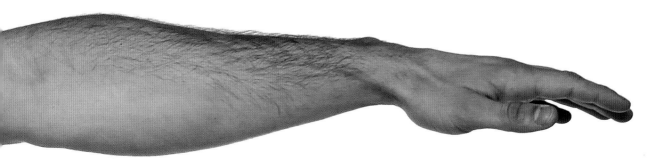

# THE
# SWIMMING LAB

# SWIM ANATOMY

**Swimming is an all-body exercise**: your trunk (core) and limbs work together to propel you through the water. While water supports your body, it also pushes against you. Efficient streamlining and sound stroke technique will transform your performance. Treat your foundation training as a laboratory: understanding each phase of your swim stroke (shown below) will help you master the first leg of the triathlon.

### KEY »

Swimming recruits all the major muscle groups, but the front crawl mainly engages your latissimus dorsi, pectorals, triceps, and biceps (shown opposite). A steady and relaxed flutter kick also uses the hip flexors, quadriceps, hamstrings, and gluteals, but more for balance than propulsion.

● PECTORALIS MAJOR ● LATISSIMUS DORSI
● GLUTEALS ● TRICEPS
● HIP FLEXORS ● BICEPS

## SWIM MECHANICS

You can use any swim stroke in a triathlon, but freestyle (front crawl) is the most efficient over long distances. Water is far denser than air and offers 1,000 times more resistance, so you need to swim as horizontally as possible to reduce drag (the water's negative force that holds you back). Some people are more buoyant than others, or have legs that sink lower, so learning how to optimize your body position in the water is essential to swimming well. Maintaining the right head position and a relaxed flutter kick will help with your body's balance and reduce drag. Then you can learn how to catch the water and power through it using your trunk and the timing of your stroke.

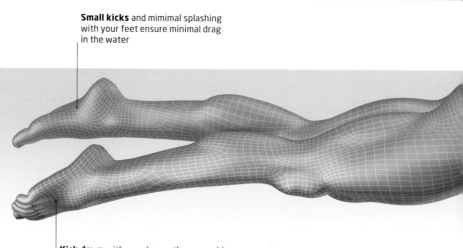

**Small kicks** and mimimal splashing with your feet ensure minimal drag in the water

**Kick down** with your leg on the same side as your "catch" arm, keeping your ankles relaxed

## ENTER AND EXTEND

The first phase is your lead arm's entry into the water. Your deltoid and shoulder muscles power the entry and reaching movement as your arm extends to full stretch.

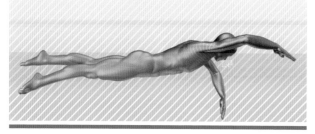

## CATCH AND PRESS

Keeping your lead arm's elbow out to the side, catch the water with your hand and press down on it to anchor yourself in the water.
As you kick down on the same side, rotating your hips and shoulders, your body is powered forwards over your hand.

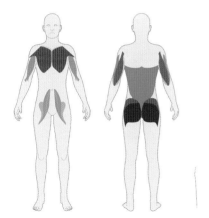

# THE KINETIC CHAIN

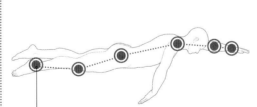

**Every element** in the chain needs to be working optimally to achieve a strong swim stroke

Your body is made to move. Its many muscles, joints, and nerves are linked together by a matrix of fascia (connective tissue) in the kinetic chain – the body's movement system. These links in the chain help you to move with great agility and coordination; a weak link, such as a sore muscle, has a knock-on effect throughout the chain, affecting performance.

**Your trunk** is where the power comes from to swim fast

**Keep your head low**, with your face in the water, to reduce drag - rotate (don't raise) your head to take a breath

**Spear the water** with your left arm while your right arm sweeps back towards your hip

**Press back** on the water to maintain your hold as your body moves forwards over your hand during the pull and sweep phase of the stroke

**Hips rotate** from side to side to help gain optimum propulsion through the water

## PULL AND SWEEP

Your forearm sweeps back against the water to pull your body forwards. At the same time, your glutes and hamstring muscles power your kick to aid your balance and propulsion in the water.

## FINISH AND RECOVER

As you pull your arm out of the water and over your head, your body is at its maximum velocity and should be as relaxed as possible, ready for another stroke. While your recovery arm comes over, your other arm sets up its catch.

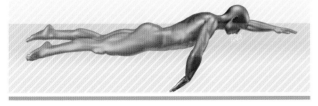

# THE EFFICIENT SWIMMER

**Essential to a successful swim** is your efficiency in the water, which you achieve in three key ways. Maintaining the correct head and body positions increases your hydrodynamics and reduces drag. A relaxed but compact leg kick further reduces drag. An effective catch gives you the solid hold on the water that allows a well-timed stroke to lever your body forwards. Structuring your foundation training around these three keys to greater efficiency will help you to become a faster swimmer.

**❝** FLEXIBLE ANKLES MAKE **EFFICIENT KICKS**, BUT TRIATHELTES **NEED STABLE ANKLES** TO SURVIVE THE RUN AND CYCLE RACES WITHOUT INJURY. **MINIMAL KICKING** THEREFORE SAVES ENERGY TO KEEP TRIATHLETES EFFICIENT IN THE WATER. **❞**

**Rotate your hips,** torso, and shoulders as one to help streamline your body throughout the stroke and propel yourself forwards

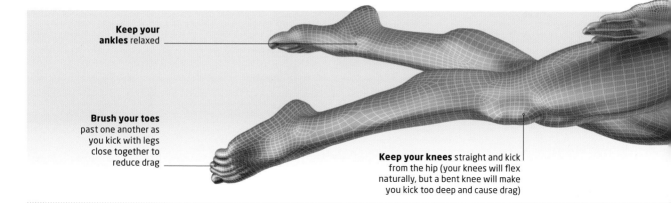

**Keep your ankles** relaxed

**Brush your toes** past one another as you kick with legs close together to reduce drag

**Keep your knees** straight and kick from the hip (your knees will flex naturally, but a bent knee will make you kick too deep and cause drag)

## LEG KICK

Swimmers tend to favour the flutter kick in competitive swimming. In the flutter kick, the legs alternate small kicks up and down, which helps with the body's rotation, balance, and overall position in the water. You get minimal propulsion from your leg kick, so don't worry about kicking hard; focus instead on your kick technique, rhythm, and timing (see pp.18–19) to complement your arm strokes.

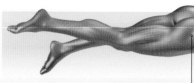

**Kick from the hips,** not from the knees

**1 Kick up** but not too high; you don't want to cause a splash as this creates drag. Instead, simply counter the down kick to keep you balanced.

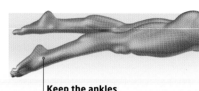

**Keep the ankles** relaxed

**2 Kicking down** at the same time as your arm on the same side sets up the catch (see pp.16–19). Keep the kick shallow to reduce drag.

## HYDRODYNAMICS

Good hydronamics is about cutting through the water more efficiently by creating minimum negative forces. Drag is the negative force that is created behind you as the water flows around your body and holds you back. Staying streamlined will reduce drag.

**A deep kick** and/or high head make your body drop low, which creates drag

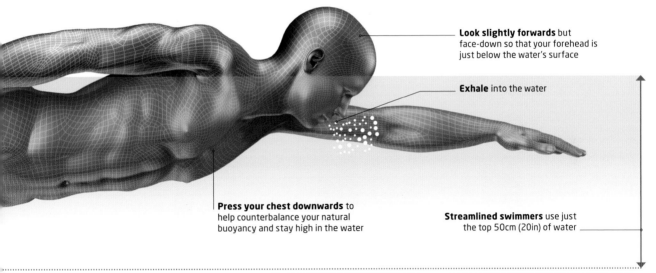

✓ **Streamlined position**
Swimming horizontally with head down, hips up, and a shallow flutter kick will create less drag.

✗ **Bad posture**
Swimming "uphill" creates immense drag because the water can't easily flow around you as you swim.

**Look slightly forwards** but face-down so that your forehead is just below the water's surface

**Exhale** into the water

**Press your chest downwards** to help counterbalance your natural buoyancy and stay high in the water

**Streamlined swimmers** use just the top 50cm (20in) of water

## BREATHING

Every action has an equal and opposite reaction. In water, lifting your head to breathe (action) makes your legs sink (reaction). Keep your head in the water when you breathe; turn your head to the side (don't raise it) during the arm's recovery, and inhale from the pocket of air there. Exhale constantly into the water through the mouth and nose to empty your lungs ready for the next breath. (See also p.19.)

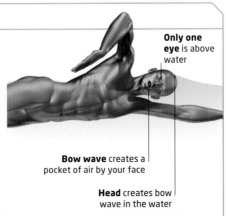

**Only one eye** is above water

**Bow wave** creates a pocket of air by your face

**Head** creates bow wave in the water

## CATCH

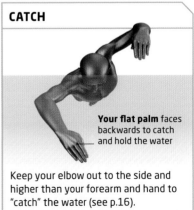

**Your flat palm** faces backwards to catch and hold the water

Keep your elbow out to the side and higher than your forearm and hand to "catch" the water (see p.16).

# THE ARM STROKE

**You need to "catch" and hold the water** to maintain your forward momentum. You do this by using your hand and forearm as an anchor. The hand does not move backwards – the body moves over the hand, your hips working with your leg kick and trunk to generate rotation and propel you forwards. Understanding the theory and mastering the technique to the four phases of your arm stroke should be the focus of your training (see pp.22–25) to transform your race performance.

❝ **EXTEND YOUR LEAD ARM** TO **FULL LENGTH** DURING ENTRY TO **MAXIMIZE YOUR REACH** AND **MOVE FURTHER FASTER** WITH EACH AND EVERY **STROKE**. ❞

## ENTER AND EXTEND

With your lead arm, spear your hand into the water in line with the same shoulder, and extend it forwards to your arm's maximum reach.

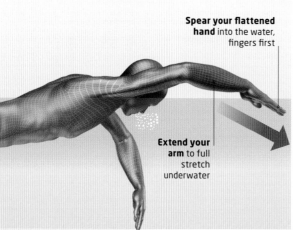

**Spear your flattened hand** into the water, fingers first

**Extend your arm** to full stretch underwater

- Rotate your body towards the same side as your lead arm, into a level position in the water (as shown above).
- This rotation of your hips and shoulders adds thrust to your lead arm's entry as you drive it into the water, fingertips first.
- Reach your lead arm forwards, extending the hand in front of you as far as possible, without over-reaching.

## CATCH

With your lead arm fully extended, you now set up the catch – the most important part of the stroke. This anchors your hand in the water, ready to lever your body forwards.

**Keep your elbow high** and bend it out to the side so that it stays higher than your forearm and hand

**Bend your hand down** so your palm faces back

- Cock your hand at the wrist (not the knuckles) so that your fingers point down and your palm faces back.
- Gently press on the water with your hand so that it starts to catch hold of the water.
- Bend your elbow to keep it higher than your wrist, and keep your wrist cocked so that your hand stays below it – this is the prime catch position. Now apply pressure to the water.

# FRONT QUADRANT SWIMMING

Efficient swimming is all about the timing of your stroke, especially at the front end of your body. Imagine the water surface as a horizontal line bissected by a vertical line at your head to create four quadrants. A successful front-quadrant swim requires one of your hands to be in one of the front two quadrants at any point in the stroke, so that you always have a leading arm. Your hands should only ever pass each other (such as when one is in the catch phase and the other is finishing the recovery phase) when they are both in front of your head.

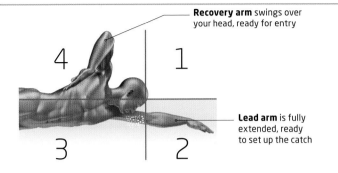

**Recovery arm** swings over your head, ready for entry

**Lead arm** is fully extended, ready to set up the catch

## PULL AND SWEEP

After the catch, press on the water with your hand to lever your body forwards and over your hand. As your shoulder passes over your hand, go from a slow pull to a fast sweep all the way to your hip.

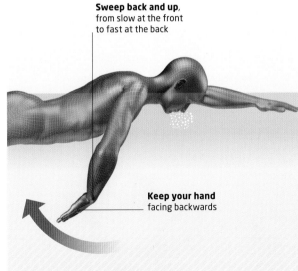

**Sweep back and up**, from slow at the front to fast at the back

**Keep your hand** facing backwards

- Keeping your elbow high to maximize the pulling power, press on the water with your hand.
- For good hydrodynamics, keep your hand facing backwards, so that you keep pushing water back behind you, not down.
- Sweep your arm back and up to the hip. To maximize the driving power of the sweep, reach your hand past your hip, with your thumb brushing your hip.

## FINISH AND RECOVERY

You finish the stroke as your hand exits the water. Lift your elbow out of the water and relax your arm to start the recovery phase. Leading with your elbow, swing your arm over your head.

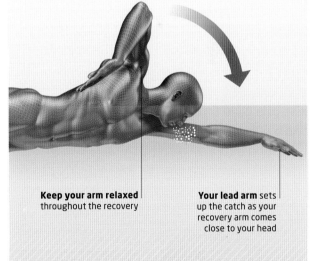

**Keep your arm relaxed** throughout the recovery

**Your lead arm** sets up the catch as your recovery arm comes close to your head

- As you pull your arm out of the water, your body is optimally rotated to your other side
- Relax your recovery arm and shoulder muscles in order to use as little energy as possible  - your other arm is leading now
- Keep your recovery elbow high so that your arm and hand fall forwards. When your elbow is above your head, drive your arm into the water to begin a new stroke

# THE STROKE CYCLE

**When you have completed** a stroke with first one arm and then the other, you have done one stroke cycle. While you are beginning to work on your stroke, you may find that you linger, or "glide", by holding your extension before setting up your catch. It is important not to rush the catch, but a longer glide does not work well for triathletes in open water. As your timing and feel for the stroke improve, your stroke cycle should speed up, with less of a glide on extension, and a quicker and smoother transition between phases.

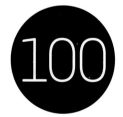

**ONE HUNDRED STROKES (50 CYCLES) PER MINUTE IS THE STROKE RATE OF ELITE ATHLETES GETTING TO THE FIRST BUOY IN AN OPEN-WATER RACE**

## STROKE CYCLE PHASES

### ENTRY AND EXTENSION
With your left arm in the catch phase, spear your right arm and shoulder into the water, and extend your arm through the water to full stretch, with the palm facing downwards.

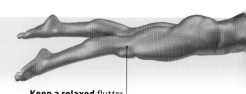

**Keep a relaxed** flutter kick between each catch

### CATCH
As you rotate to your right side and swing your left arm over your head, set up the catch with your right arm: keep your elbow out to the side and higher than your forearm and hand. Now you are ready for the press, kick, and counter-rotation that propel you forwards.

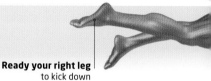

**Rotate your hips, shoulders, and torso** to the right as you pull your left arm up and over

**Ready your right leg** to kick down

### PULL AND SWEEP
As you simultaneously press the water, kick down and rotate back towards your left side, steadily pull on the water with your right hand, palm facing back. Then sweep your arm towards your hip, going from slow to fast to maintain your hold on the water.

**Flutter kick** between each catch

### FINISH
When your right hand finishes its stroke and leaves the water, your body is at full stretch and maximum velocity. If you have a fast stroke rate, your hand might flick water as it exits. When you race in open water, the finish is when you look to sight the next buoy (see pp.30-31).

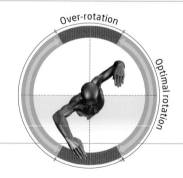

Over-rotation

Optimal rotation

### RECOVERY
As your right hand exits the water, relax and pull your arm up, leading with your elbow. When your elbow swings over your head, start to reach forward, ready to begin another stroke cycle.

**Rotate your shoulders, torso, and hips** as one to an angle of 45-60 degrees; the more buoyant you are, the less you will need to rotate. Over-rotation reduces your power and efficiency.

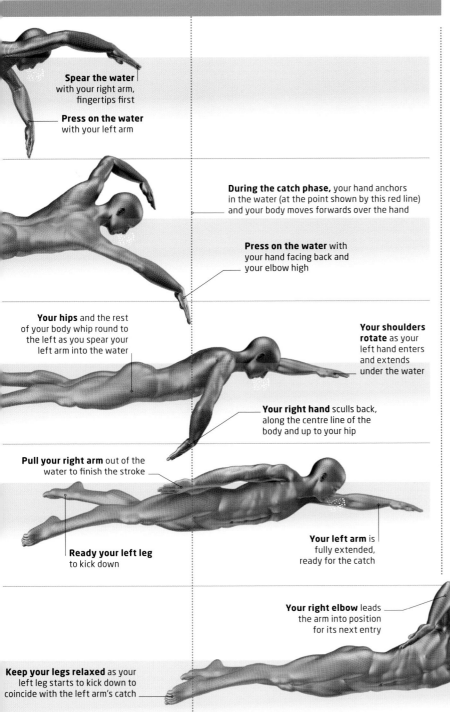

**Spear the water** with your right arm, fingertips first

**Press on the water** with your left arm

**During the catch phase,** your hand anchors in the water (at the point shown by this red line) and your body moves forwards over the hand

**Press on the water** with your hand facing back and your elbow high

**Your hips** and the rest of your body whip round to the left as you spear your left arm into the water

**Your shoulders rotate** as your left hand enters and extends under the water

**Your right hand** sculls back, along the centre line of the body and up to your hip

**Pull your right arm** out of the water to finish the stroke

**Ready your left leg** to kick down

**Your left arm** is fully extended, ready for the catch

**Your right elbow** leads the arm into position for its next entry

**Keep your legs relaxed** as your left leg starts to kick down to coincide with the left arm's catch

**Set up the catch** with your left arm when your right arm reaches your head

## TIMING

### KICKS PER CYCLE

The most energy-efficient kick is the two-beat kick (two kicks per arm cycle), although some swimmers use a four- or six-beat kick to help balance their bodies. The key to fast swimming is timing. The timing of your downward kick should match the timing of your hand on the same side: once you have set up the catch and start to apply pressure on the water with your hand, you simultaneously kick down and rotate on the same side.

**" AFTER THE FIRST BUOY,** THE STROKE RATE OF **ELITE ATHLETES** SLOWS SLIGHTLY AND SETTLES AT ABOUT **75-80 STROKES** (40 ARM CYCLES) PER MINUTE. **"**

### BREATHS PER CYCLE

Different swimmers employ different breathing tactics. The less you turn your head to breathe, the less you disrupt your hydrodynamics. Even so, you need oxygen, so in a race it is fine to use whichever breathing technique you are comfortable with. In training, try to use bilateral breathing: breathing to both sides (every three, five, or seven strokes) develops more balanced muscle use.

# WARMING UP

**Swimming warm-ups** are an essential part of effective training. Moving and stretching the muscles before getting into the water, followed by a familiar warm-up routine, help enhance performance and prevent injury.

## DRY-LAND WARM-UP

The aim of a dry-land warm-up is to activate your body and get the blood flowing to the key muscles before you set foot in the water. It should be performed for between 5 and 10 minutes before you start swimming.

**1 VISUALIZATION** Stand looking out at the pool or water you are about to swim in. Visualize your extension and catch (see pp.16-19), imagining what each movement will feel like as you travel through the water, and move your arms accordingly. Continue visualizing your swim through the water as you move your arms through the rest of the stroke cycle 10 times.

Keep your rotating arm straight

Your bicep should brush your ear

**2 VERTICAL ARM SWING** Holding both arms straight out in front of your chest, drop your right arm and rotate it in a full circle 10 times. Repeat with your left arm, then rotate each arm backwards 10 times.

# BACKSTROKE

A great swim warm-up, backstroke balances out the muscles that are used most in front crawl by working the antagonist muscle groups (the muscles that contract as their counterparts relax). It's also a calming way to start the swim: your face is out of the water, so there's no need to worry about breathing patterns.

Lie on your back with your arms at your sides. Flutter kick your legs. Raise your arm out of the water and rotate it back above your head in line with your shoulder. Gently bring it down into the water (simultaneously starting the next stroke with your other arm) and sweep it back to your side to finish one revolution. Complete 200-400m (220-440yd) at a steady pace.

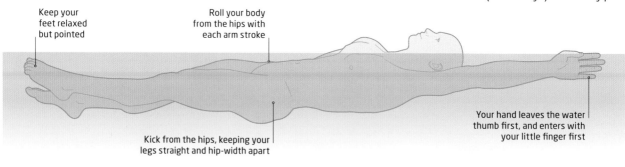

Keep your feet relaxed but pointed

Roll your body from the hips with each arm stroke

Kick from the hips, keeping your legs straight and hip-width apart

Your hand leaves the water thumb first, and enters with your little finger first

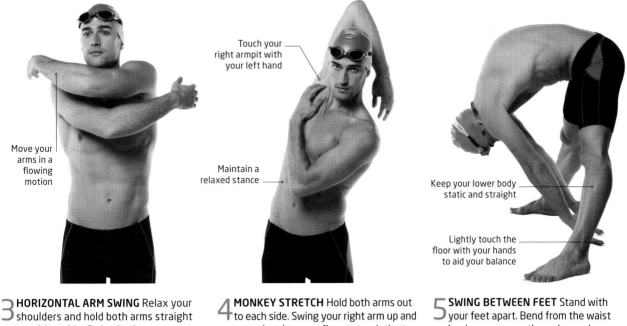

Move your arms in a flowing motion

Touch your right armpit with your left hand

Maintain a relaxed stance

Keep your lower body static and straight

Lightly touch the floor with your hands to aid your balance

**3 HORIZONTAL ARM SWING** Relax your shoulders and hold both arms straight out to either side. Swing both arms in across your chest to hug yourself, reaching around your back to touch your shoulder blades. Repeat 10 times.

**4 MONKEY STRETCH** Hold both arms out to each side. Swing your right arm up and over your head so your fingers touch the top of your spine. At the same time, swing your left arm up to touch your opposite armpit. Repeat 10 times, alternating arms.

**5 SWING BETWEEN FEET** Stand with your feet apart. Bend from the waist and swing your arms through your legs, out in front of you, and back through your legs. Swing your upper body back to the start position. Repeat 10 times.

# FRONT SCULLING

This drill involves the back-and-forth movement of the hands through the water in a U-shape. Front sculling is an excellent way to increase your feel for the water and make your hand movements more effective.

Start on your front, with your face in the water and your arms stretched in front of you. Bring your elbows slightly out to the sides, with your palms facing down. Hinge from the elbow, scoop your arms down through the water in a U-shape, and back again. Keep your elbows in front of your shoulders and slightly bent. Hold your head out of the water to elongate the front of your body. Kick deeply from your hips. Complete four 50m (55yd) sets with a 10-second rest between each.

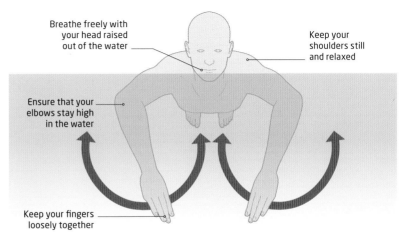

Breathe freely with your head raised out of the water

Keep your shoulders still and relaxed

Ensure that your elbows stay high in the water

Keep your fingers loosely together

# SWIM DRILLS

**A sequence of simple drills** can work wonders at helping to improve your stroke technique and balance, efficiency in the water, and overall performance. Forget about speed for now while you get to grips with these drills; focus on technique to begin with and your time will improve in due course.

## BUILD YOUR STROKE

These drills take you step by step through each element of the freestyle stroke, building on each aspect until you're swimming a complete stroke. Assess your performance and prioritize those drills that target your weaknesses. Practise them in sequence and don't move on until you've mastered each one.

## 01 HEAD ROTATION DRILL

Good breathing technique is as important as your catch at keeping you efficient in the water. Practise breathing on both sides so that you can apply bilateral breathing to your stroke.

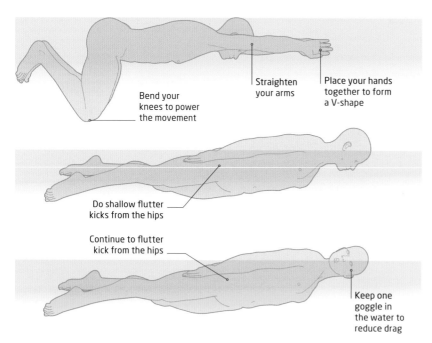

Straighten your arms

Place your hands together to form a V-shape

Bend your knees to power the movement

Do shallow flutter kicks from the hips

Continue to flutter kick from the hips

Keep one goggle in the water to reduce drag

**KIT BOX: FINS**

Swimming fins can be a useful practice prop: they increase your sensitivity to the water, help you stay in a streamlined position, strengthen your leg muscles, and give your kick more power so you can focus on perfecting other aspects of your stroke.

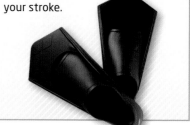

❝ RELAXATION IS KEY WHEN LEARNING TO **BREATHE CORRECTLY**. SNATCHING FOR AIR WILL **DISRUPT YOUR RHYTHM**. ❞

1 Take a deep breath and duck your head beneath the water. Position both feet on the wall behind you and push off strongly with arms stretched straight out in front of you. This is called a torpedo push-off.

2 Kick your legs to propel yourself forward and rotate onto one side. Bring your arms to your sides and keep them straight against your body. Find a relaxed rhythm with your kicking.

3 Rotate your head to breathe, tilting it back in the water. Then rotate your head back into the water, and slowly exhale. Continue to swim forwards for 25m (30yd), rotating and tilting your head to breathe whenever you need to, then roll onto your other side and repeat for 25m. Repeat for a further 25m on each side.

## 02 **FULL BODY** ROTATION DRILL

This drill introduces you to the kick-rotation movement that will propel your body through the water during freestyle. Drive the rotation with your hips, aided by a carefully timed kick.

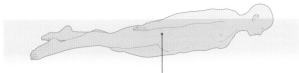

Do shallow flutter kicks from your hips

1 Perform the torpedo push-off. Before you start to slow, bring your arms to your sides. Start to flutter kick. Find your balance in the water and maintain a steady kicking rhythm, counting each time you kick down. Breathe when necessary.

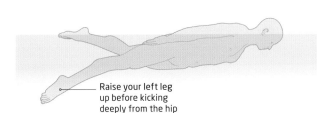

Raise your left leg up before kicking deeply from the hip

2 After six kicks, kick down with your left leg and twist your hips and shoulders to the left, rotating your whole body face-down through the water. Continue flutter kicking on your left side. Rotate and tilt your head to breathe when necessary.

Raise your right leg up in preparation for kicking

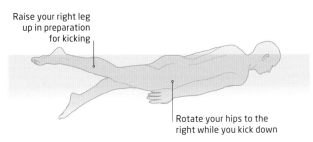

Rotate your hips to the right while you kick down

3 After six kicks, kick down with your right leg and twist your hips to the right, rotating your whole body face-down through the water. Repeat the rotation on alternate sides every six kicks for 100m (110yd). Stay relaxed and take breaths when necessary.

## 03 **RECOVERY** ARM DRILL

Once you have mastered your breathing technique and body rotation, you can start thinking about your arms. This drill focuses on positioning your recovery arm correctly.

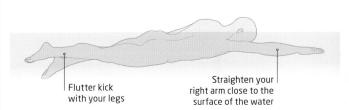

Flutter kick with your legs

Straighten your right arm close to the surface of the water

1 Perform the torpedo push-off. Roll onto your right side, bringing your left arm to your side and leaving your right arm extended in front of you. Look down but forwards. Maintain a relaxed kicking rhythm and breathe when needed.

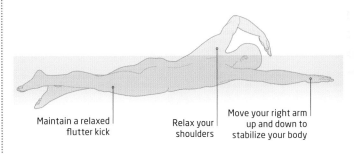

Maintain a relaxed flutter kick

Relax your shoulders

Move your right arm up and down to stabilize your body

2 Bring your left "recovery" arm out of the water, elbow first. As you swing your arm over your head, allow your forearm to hinge down and point your hand towards the water. Pause in this position before bringing your arm back to your side.

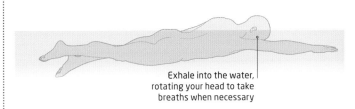

Exhale into the water, rotating your head to take breaths when necessary

3 Repeat your left arm's recovery arm raise and pause every six kicks for 25m (30yd). Stay relaxed and take breaths when necessary. Repeat on your right side for 25m. Repeat for a further 25m on each side.

# 04 **CATCH ARM** DRILL

During the stroke cycle (see pp.18-19), your leading arm will perform the "catch", anchoring your body in the water as your hip rotation propels you through the water. This drill will give you a feel for the correct catch arm position.

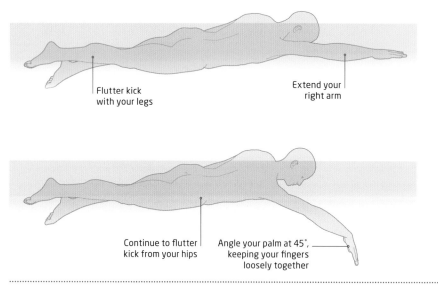

Flutter kick with your legs

Extend your right arm

Continue to flutter kick from your hips

Angle your palm at 45°, keeping your fingers loosely together

**1** Torpedo push off, then roll onto your right side, bringing your left arm down to your side and leaving your right arm extended in front of you. Look down towards the bottom of the pool and flutter kick your legs.

**2** Cock your hand down at the wrist and bend your elbow out to the side, higher than your forearm and hand. This is the catch position. Pause before extending your arm back in front of you. Repeat the catch and pause every six kicks for 25m (30yd). Take breaths when necessary. Repeat on your left side for 25m. Repeat for a further 25m on each side.

# 05 **FULL STROKE** DRILL

This drill sees you practise your first full freestyle stroke. It incorporates every aspect of the stroke that you've already mastered, and requires you to follow through the arm movements and focus on the timing of each element.

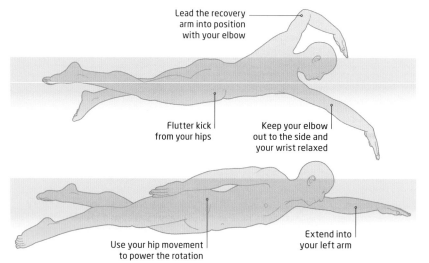

Lead the recovery arm into position with your elbow

Flutter kick from your hips

Keep your elbow out to the side and your wrist relaxed

Use your hip movement to power the rotation

Extend into your left arm

**1** Torpedo push off, then roll onto your right side, bringing your left arm to your side and leaving your right arm extended in front. Look down and flutter kick your legs. Bring your left arm up to the recovery position, simultaneously setting up the catch with your right arm. Pause with both arms in position.

**2** Kick down with your right leg and press down on the water with your right hand, then sweep your arm back to your hips. Drive your left arm into the water as you rotate your body on to your left side. Kick six times before repeating the drill on your right side. Repeat on alternate sides every six kicks for 100m (110yd).

# 06 **STROKE TIMING** DRILL

Building on the previous drill, this exercise focuses on practising the full stroke cycle – this time on both sides one after the other, with breathing integrated into the stroke.

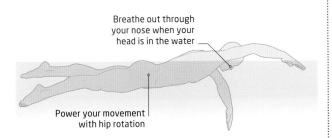

Breathe out through your nose when your head is in the water

Power your movement with hip rotation

1 Torpedo push off and assume the start position for the full stroke drill, on your left side with your right arm at your side and your left arm extended. Complete a stroke on your left side, pausing with your arms in position. Then, repeat on your right side.

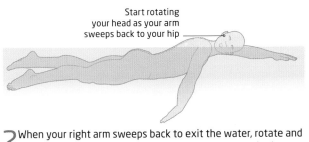

Start rotating your head as your arm sweeps back to your hip

2 When your right arm sweeps back to exit the water, rotate and tilt your head to breathe. Complete the stroke. Kick six times before repeating the drill. Repeat every six kicks for 100m (110yd).

# 07 **THREE STROKE** DRILL

Having mastered the full stroke cycle with both arms, it's time to combine them to complete three full strokes, one after another. Remember to pause in the correct catch/recovery position.

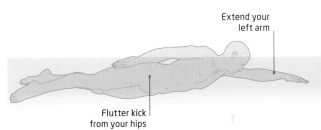

Extend your left arm

Flutter kick from your hips

1 Torpedo push off and assume the start position for the full stroke drill, on your left side with your right arm at your side and your left arm extended. Complete a stroke on your left side, right side, and left side again.

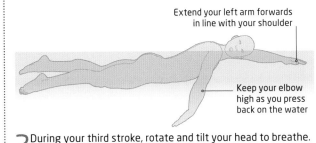

Extend your left arm forwards in line with your shoulder

Keep your elbow high as you press back on the water

2 During your third stroke, rotate and tilt your head to breathe. Kick six times before repeating the drill. Repeat every six kicks for 100m (110yd).

# 08 **SEVEN STROKE** DRILL

This drill repeats the previous one, but increases the number of arm strokes you perform. Once you can complete this extended exercise smoothly, you're ready to move on to swimming lengths freestyle, without pausing during catch/recovery.

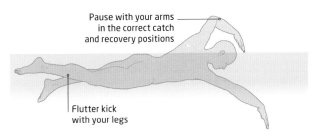

Pause with your arms in the correct catch and recovery positions

Flutter kick with your legs

1 Repeat the previous drill, this time completing seven full strokes. Breathe on every third stroke. Kick six times before repeating the drill. Repeat every six kicks for 100m (110yd).

# SWIM SESSIONS

**While some elite athletes** train in the pool six or seven times a week and swim 5,000-8,000m (3-5 miles) each session, those new to swimming should focus on improving technique and efficiency before looking to swim further or faster. Training at the different levels of intensity shown below will allow you to target different aspects of your fitness and technique. Beginning with three sessions a week, most of your sessions should be at Levels 1 and 2, with a smaller proportion of higher-level sessions. Using swimming aids can also help develop your efficiency and strength.

## SWIMMING AIDS

A pull buoy between the thighs makes your legs float so you can focus on developing arm power. Small hand paddles improve your "hold" of the water; large paddles increase resistance to strengthen arms. (See p.22 for fins.)

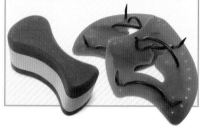

## TRAINING LEVELS 1-5

### 1 EASY

Calm swimming to allow you to work on the catch during the pause phase, re-emphasizing its importance in your stroke technique.

**TARGET:** 50-60 per cent of maximum heart rate (HR max).

**MAIN SET:** Complete the following in sequence, pausing on catch for the first 25m (27yd) of each repetition. Have the swimming aids accessible to minimize stoppage time.
- Steady pace front crawl x 100m (110yd)
- Pull buoy between legs x 100m (110yd)
- Paddles on hands x 100m (110yd)
- Pull buoy and paddles x 100m (110yd)
- Pull buoy and band round ankles x 100m (110yd)

**RECOVERY:** At the end of each 100m (110yd), pause and take 3-5 breaths.

**PROGRESSION:** Increase by 100m (110yd) each week.

**BENEFITS:** The relaxed swim helps you to focus on technical elements.

### 2 TEMPO

Focuses on the technical side of the swim, including bringing more rhythm into your stroke.

**TARGET:** 60-70 per cent of HR max.

**MAIN SET:** Complete in sequence, then alternate and repeat to 1,000m (1,100yd) total. Have the swim aids accessible to minimize stoppage time.
- Steady pace front crawl x 200m (220yd)
- Steady pace front crawl with fins and paddles x 200m (220yd)

**RECOVERY:** At the end of each 200m (220yd), pause while you put on/take off the swimming aids.

**PROGRESSION:** Aim to increase the distance by 10 per cent, but only once you've mastered the stroke mechanics; being technically perfect will enable faster swimming later.

**BENEFITS:** Swimming with aids and then without increases sensory perception; fins and paddles emphasize the importance of the catch and kick, especially once they're removed.

### 3 THRESHOLD

Race-pace sequence to build speed. Swimming at your threshold will feel good for a few lengths; however, you must maintain good stroke mechanics even as you tire.

**TARGET:** 70-85 per cent of HR max.

**MAIN SET:** Select and complete one of these sets depending on your level of fitness and swimming ability.
- Front crawl 200m (220yd) race pace swim, OR
- Front crawl 400m (440yd) race pace swim

**RECOVERY:** Take half of your swim set time (e.g. 6 mins swim = 3 mins recovery) for either passive (resting) recovery or active (backstroke) recovery.

**PROGRESSION:** As your fitness improves, double the swim distance to 2 x 200m (220yd) or 2 x 400m (440yd), or reduce your recovery time.

**BENEFITS:** Learning about your personal "race pace" and how you manage exertion is key to success; starting a race too fast usually ends in failure.

## SAMPLE SESSION

Using a sample session from Level 2, this table shows how to structure the session in four parts, starting with a warm-up. Adapt your sets to your needs - push yourself beyond your comfort zone, but don't overdo it and risk injury. Gradually increase distance or duration as your fitness improves.
*For a sample foundation programme of weekly sessions, see pp.122-123.*

| L2 SESSION | SAMPLE ACTIVITY |
|---|---|
| WARM-UP | Backstroke 200-400m (220-440yd): complements front crawl, increases your heart rate, and focuses the mind |
| PRE-MAIN DRILL SET | Drill sets 100m (110yd) each: increases your feel of the water; improves catch and thrust in strokes |
| MAIN SET | Complete main set for Level 2 (see below); increase distance or duration as your fitness improves |
| COOL-DOWN | Front crawl/backstroke 200-400m (220-440yd): winds body down slowly, reducing risk of injury |

## 4 vVO2 MAX

Intense pace to increase your vVO2 max (the speed at which your body's oxygen consumption peaks) at your race-start swim speed. Starting well and settling back into a sustainable pace will help your overall race time.

**TARGET:** 85-96 per cent of HR max.

**MAIN SET:** Front crawl 6 x 100-150m (110-165yd), hard.

**RECOVERY:** The first time you do this, just make sure you feel recovered before you go again. Then match your recovery time to the time of the set.

**PROGRESSION:** Gradually increase the number of repetitions (reps) until the set matches the distance to your first race buoy; or include race-pace swimming to mimic a race scenario. Do not decrease recovery time; it can affect your stroke.

**BENEFITS:** Push harder and your workout will become anaerobic (see pp.160-161), increasing your lactate tolerance (to reduce muscle soreness), and helping you dissipate lactate when you settle back to race pace or below.

## 5 MAXIMAL

A maximum-pace swim set, this session aims to improve sprinting ability and swimming power by focusing on your stroke quality at speed.

**TARGET:** 96-100 per cent of HR max.

**MAIN SET:** Front crawl 10 x 25-50m (28-55yd), maximum pace.

**RECOVERY:** Take double the recovery time for each length (e.g. 20 seconds to swim = 40 seconds to rest).

**PROGRESSION:** Increase the distance of each sprint, although don't sprint for more than 150-200m (165-220yd). Alternatively, increase the number of reps in each set. Retain the recovery time as this ensures efficiency.

**BENEFITS:** By focusing on the catch of each and every stroke and setting it up correctly, you will maximize efficiency and increase swim power. Remember to increase the speed of your recovery arm and kick a little harder to go faster.

For more details on how Levels 1-5 target physiology and fitness, see pp.160-161.

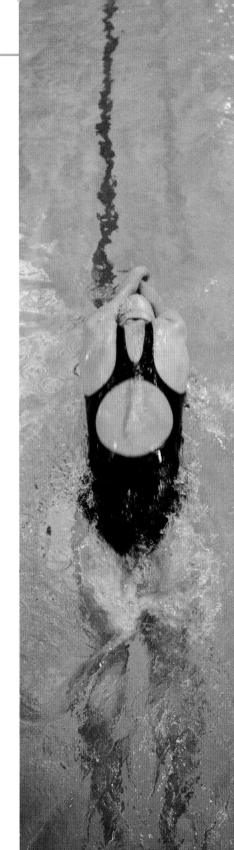

# ASSESSING YOUR SWIM FITNESS

**Swimming is a non-weight-bearing** discipline, but you are still up against water, which is a thousand times denser than air. Your preparation will be most efficient if you have an accurate idea of how fit you are before you start training.

## Q WHAT'S THE FIRST STEP?

**A** Before embarking on any form of strenuous exercise, the smart move is to begin with a general health check. If you have any existing medical conditions ask your doctor how they will affect your training. Even if you are completely well, different body types and ages may require different training regimes.

## Q WHAT ARE THE MAIN RISK FACTORS?

**A** You need to be particularly mindful of your blood pressure and cholesterol levels, and get yourself tested for iron deficiency and diabetes. If you have high blood pressure, heavy exercise can damage the veins and arteries, while high cholesterol impedes bloodflow to your heart. Iron helps the blood to carry oxygen to the muscles, so you need to be sure you have enough of this vital mineral. Diabetes needn't prevent you from training, but it does affect the regulation of blood sugar levels (see pp.90-91).

## Q HOW DO I MEASURE MY GENERAL FITNESS?

**A** Your fitness will greatly impact your swimming performance. There are some simple fitness tests you can do yourself. First, find your resting heart rate (see opposite) and check it against the chart on p.158. Your resting heart rate is a good indicator of your general fitness and is the baseline from which you will work. Next, calculate your VO2 max. One of the oldest fitness indices, VO2 max measures the volume (V) of oxygen ($O_2$) that you are able to take in and use when you are exercising at optimum (maximum) rates (see pp.78-79 for further details).

## Q HOW DO I MEASURE MY SWIM FITNESS?

**A** Since swimming is easy on the joints, fitness concerns will be mainly about heart rates and endurance. The tests here should give you a good idea of your swim fitness so you can start training at the right level. Retest yourself every 8-12 weeks.

---

### DO A 400 M / 400-YARD TEST

You can do this in any pool, but a 25m or 28-yard pool makes distance calculations easy. You will need to do 16 lengths a pool this size.

#### WHAT TO DO

1 **Warm-up** You must do this if you want to swim well in the test (see the swim warm-up on pp.20-21).

2 **Dive** If you're a beginner, you may prefer a push start. Be consistent and use the same dive or push start whenever you repeat the test.

3 **Swim 200m / 220 yards** Build up to just above the pace you are aiming for in the test. Allow yourself to recover before the main swim.

4 **Swim 400m / 440 yards** Swim at a pace you can sustain for the whole test, as this will boost stamina.

#### WHAT TO RECORD
• **Swim time and stroke count** This assessment is best done with a friend timing you, recording your stroke count (strokes per length) over four 100m / 110-yard "splits" (sections) of your swim. To do the test on your own, either record your overall time or press "split" on your GPS watch (see p.32) every 100m / 110 yards.

• **Stroke count** How many arm strokes do you take per length? Record this every 100m /110 yards.

#### HOW DO YOU RATE?
Elite swimmers complete this test in under 4 minutes 30 seconds, while some top age-group athletes will do it in about 8 minutes. Remember not to swim at your "race pace" but at around your Level 4 pace (see pp.26-27), making it quite challenging near the end.

## FIND YOUR RESTING HEART RATE

This test measures the rate at which your heart beats when you haven't been exerting yourself. Ideally you should do it first thing in the morning before you get up. In general, the lower the rate, the fitter you are (see p.158).

Note that if you are dehydrated, your heart rate may go up by 7.5 per cent. It is also likely to rise if you are stressed or emotional, perhaps by 10–20 per cent. For an accurate resting heart rate, you should be hydrated, calm, and relaxed.

A higher than usual resting heart rate can be sign of illness; if your rate is high, decide whether to rest or lower the intensity or duration of training until your heart rate returns to normal.

### WHAT TO DO

Lie down with a watch or clock within easy reach and clearly visible. Carefully locate the pulse at your neck or wrist, then count the number of beats in one minute, remaining as still as you can.

## MEASURE YOUR TRAINING: THE RPE SCALE

The Rate of Perceived Exertion (RPE) scale measures the intensity of exercise. In this book, it is correlated to heart rate zones (see below). The RPE scale rates exercise intensity from 1 to 10. An RPE of 1 puts minimal strain on the body, while an RPE of 10 is your maximum effort. An easy workout in the pool should be about RPE 3–4, or 60–70 per cent of your maximum heart rate.

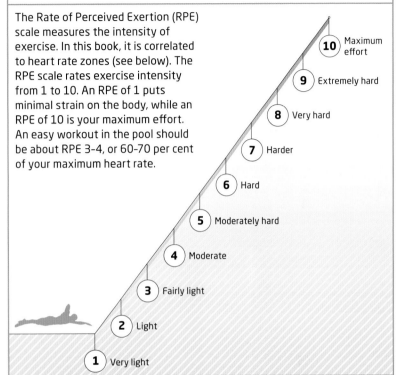

10 Maximum effort
9 Extremely hard
8 Very hard
7 Harder
6 Hard
5 Moderately hard
4 Moderate
3 Fairly light
2 Light
1 Very light

## CALCULATE YOUR WORKING HEART RATE AND HEART RATE ZONES

Your heart rate is a good indicator of how hard your body is working. The more you exercise, the more oxygen your muscles need, so your heart beats faster to pump oxygenated blood around the body. Different levels of training involve specific heart rate "zones" - percentage ranges of your working heart rate.

### WHAT TO DO

To calculate your working heart rate, subtract your age from 220. This is your maximum heart rate. Next, subtract your resting heart rate from this number. You can then use your working heart rate to work out the ideal heart rate zones for your training levels.

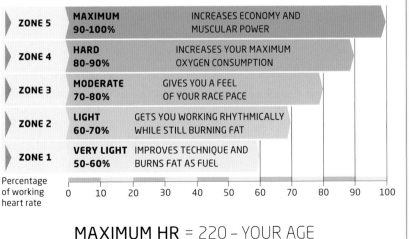

| | | |
|---|---|---|
| ZONE 5 | MAXIMUM 90–100% | INCREASES ECONOMY AND MUSCULAR POWER |
| ZONE 4 | HARD 80–90% | INCREASES YOUR MAXIMUM OXYGEN CONSUMPTION |
| ZONE 3 | MODERATE 70–80% | GIVES YOU A FEEL OF YOUR RACE PACE |
| ZONE 2 | LIGHT 60–70% | GETS YOU WORKING RHYTHMICALLY WHILE STILL BURNING FAT |
| ZONE 1 | VERY LIGHT 50–60% | IMPROVES TECHNIQUE AND BURNS FAT AS FUEL |

Percentage of working heart rate: 0 10 20 30 40 50 60 70 80 90 100

MAXIMUM HR = 220 – YOUR AGE
WORKING HR = MAXIMUM HR – RESTING HR

# OPEN-WATER SWIMMING

**With waves, currents,** and no lanes to guide you, open-water swimming is very different from training in a pool, so it pays to be prepared. Even at elite level, some athletes panic, so do not be disheartened if you find the open water daunting. Accept the external elements so you can focus on those you have control over, such as your breathing and sighting. With practice and positive mental attitude, all the training and preparation will pay off and any panic will subside with experience.

> **" RENT A WETSUIT** BEFORE YOU BUY. A WELL-FITTING WETSUIT **REDUCES AVERAGE HEART RATE BY AROUND 10%**, WHICH CAN BENEFIT YOUR OVERALL RACE. **"**

## YOUR ROUTE TO SUCCESS

### SIGHTING

Sighting is about looking where you are going in open water. As your body moves forward and your recovery arm extends to take the next stroke, lift your head very slightly, just breaking the surface of the water with your eyes but high enough to see over any swell or waves, and look forward. You need to work this into the timing of your stroke, and should sight roughly every 3-6 strokes to ensure you are on course. Once you are confident that your stroke is balanced and you are swimming in a straight line, you can sight less often.

### ROUNDING BUSY BUOYS

This is a lesson in toughness and learning not to concede water to your fellow athletes: in your first few races, remain on the outside of the swim pack or towards the back. You will lose time using this tactic, but there is no swimming technique to help you round buoys in the middle of the pack - you just have to keep moving forward and keep your head above water. With experience and confidence, you will become more capable of holding your place closer to the front and still swim strongly around the buoys.

### DRAFTING

There is an art to swimming directly behind or next to another swimmer, so practise in advance. A good technique can make you more efficient in your swim. The key is to choose another swimmer who is slightly faster than you, and benefit from swimming in their wake, with your extended arm at their hip or feet level. You do not want to disrupt their stroke or hit their feet, so a steady speed is important, as well as holding your nerve.

## IN THE PACK

- Indoors or out, going through a swim warm-up (see pp.20–21) will help you to feel calm, focused, and ready to race
- Be respectful of other swimmers, but don't concede your water
- Believe in yourself and your training; stay focused to maintain good stroke mechanics, and adapt where necessary
- Sight the buoys every 3-6 strokes

## GETTING USED TO YOUR WETSUIT

A well-fitting wetsuit (see pp.32–33) will feel tight around the neck and chest, almost restrictive. Familiarize yourself with wearing the wetsuit and putting it on before you actually race in it. While it will make you more buoyant in the water, it will also limit your stroke a little, and so you will need to adapt to work with that: do a training session in your wetsuit, learning to balance and feel your stroke while wearing it.

**Practise** zipping and unzipping your wetsuit to help with a speedy transition when you race

## GETTING OUT OF TROUBLE

Sometimes you will find yourself caught between other swimmers who disrupt your stroke and swimming. To get out of this situation, drop back slightly and roll over their hips and legs, with your back to their hips to avoid being kicked in the stomach and winded. Once you are over and free, continue at your own race speed.

## IT'S NOT YOU

It doesn't always matter how prepared you are - some things will still go awry. There are very few intentional acts of foul play during races; it is more often a case of individuals seeking their own clear water and you being caught up in the moment. Try not to take matters personally. Remain focused on finishing the swim and the rest of the race ahead.

## MAKING A CLEAN EXIT

When you are about 100m (330ft) from the swim exit, start to increase your leg kick slightly. This will get the blood flowing more to your legs from your upper body, and will help make the run to your first transition (T1) a little easier. Keep swimming for as long as possible - a few strokes after your fingers, in the catch position, first touch the bottom. Once you stand, move swiftly to the transition area, unzipping your wetsuit and pulling your arms out as you make your way towards T1 (see pp.34–35). You will then only need to remove the bottom half of the wetsuit as you get ready for the next discipline.

# WHAT TO WEAR

**Whether you wear** a wetsuit or a tri suit for the race, it needs to be comfortable. Always check International Triathlon Union (ITU) rules about the use of wetsuits, as regulations vary depending on the temperature of the water and whether the race is taking place in a pool or open water. A tri suit can be worn for the entire race and will save valuable time in transition (T1 and T2), when you switch from the swim to the bike and run.

> **WATER CONDUCTS HEAT AWAY FROM THE BODY 25–40 TIMES FASTER THAN AIR, SO MAKE SURE THAT YOU HAVE ADEQUATE INSULATION IN COLDER WATER.**

### Q | WHAT SHOULD I WEAR FOR TRAINING?

**A** If the water is temperate, you can wear your regular swimming costume or trunks for training. Your outfit needs to be tight to reduce drag (although experienced swimmers sometimes wear "drag shorts" to build up strength and water resistance). A swim hat reduces drag from hair and is more hygienic. When buying new goggles, check the fit by pressing them into your eye sockets; if they immediately fall off without the band to keep them on, they may leak.

### Q | WHAT SHOULD I WEAR IN COLD WATER?

**A** If training in cold water, a full-length wetsuit with sleeves is your best option. Wetsuits work by retaining a small layer of water against your skin, so a good fit is crucial. If the suit is too loose, it will let in water and slow you down. If you are a weaker swimmer, try a suit with a larger, or thicker, buoyancy panel. In very cold water, wear a warm neoprene hat under your swim hat. Rinse your wesuit with clean water after use and dry it flat.

### Q | WHAT SHOULD I WEAR IN WARM WATER?

**A** A swimskin is a thinner, non-buoyant alternative to a wetsuit; it compresses your body and thus reduces your drag. You can wear your tri suit under your swimskin in a warm-water or non-wetsuit race, but you will be disqualified if you wear sleeves that cover your shoulders.

### Q | WHAT CAN I WEAR FOR THE WHOLE TRIATHLON?

**A** A tri suit is an all-purpose garment that you can wear for every stage of the race.

Choose a tri suit made from quick-drying fabric that "wicks" water away from the skin (see p.55). Tri suits come in either one- or two-piece styles and can be worn under a wetsuit for longer-distance triathlons or in cold-water races.

### Q | WHAT ELSE DO I NEED?

**A** Apply water-resistant sunscreen (avoiding the eyes). Female swimmers may choose to wear a sports bra under the suit. It should be supportive enough for the run but not too heavy to dry quickly. Put lubricant on your neck, wrists, and ankles before you put your wetsuit on: this will minimize chafing and speed up removal in T1 (pp.34–35).

---

### GLOBAL POSITIONING SYSTEM (GPS) WATCH

A GPS watch can be useful for all legs of the triathlon. It provides data on your heart rate and speed that you can then upload onto your online training plan. Depending on the model, you can use the watch to track laps and strokes, but not all models are suitable for open-water swims: check before you buy. Any gadget can malfunction, so make sure you know how to train without one and check your RPE (see p.29).

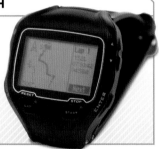

# WETSUITS

Wetsuits should be close-fitting and have enough stretch to allow good arm and shoulder mobility. Thicker wetsuits may be more buoyant, but they are not ideal for faster swimmers as they may lift the body too high in the water.

# TRI SUITS

Wearing a tri suit for the whole race will help you save precious time on the day. Choose a tri suit in a quick-drying fabric with a small chamois pad (see p.54) to make the cycling and running stages more comfortable.

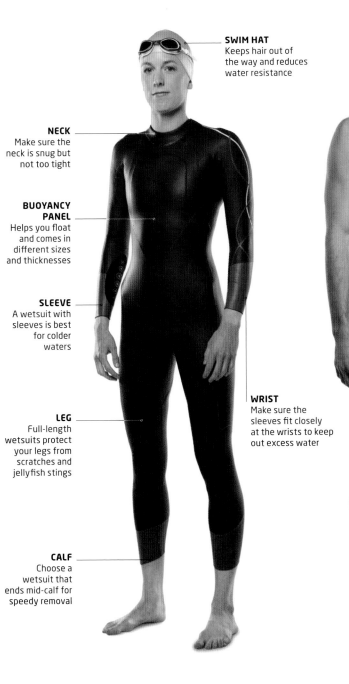

**SWIM HAT**
Keeps hair out of the way and reduces water resistance

**NECK**
Make sure the neck is snug but not too tight

**BUOYANCY PANEL**
Helps you float and comes in different sizes and thicknesses

**SLEEVE**
A wetsuit with sleeves is best for colder waters

**LEG**
Full-length wetsuits protect your legs from scratches and jellyfish stings

**WRIST**
Make sure the sleeves fit closely at the wrists to keep out excess water

**CALF**
Choose a wetsuit that ends mid-calf for speedy removal

**GOGGLES**
Wear tinted goggles in open water to reduce glare

**FABRIC**
Choose a suit made from moisture-wicking fabric to conduct sweat away from the skin

**CHAMOIS PAD**
The pad is thinner than a regular bike-short chamois, as thick, wet padding can be uncomfortable for faster runners (or during shorter runs)

**LEG**
A snug fit is important, but avoid suits that restrict circulation or leave red marks on the legs

# TRANSITION ONE (T1)

**The best way to achieve** a successful transition is to plan ahead. Make a checklist of essential equipment and practise moving from the water to the bike as part of your weekly training routine. Mastering the key skills of transition before the race will save you valuable time on the day.

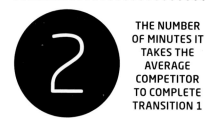

**2** THE NUMBER OF MINUTES IT TAKES THE AVERAGE COMPETITOR TO COMPLETE TRANSITION 1

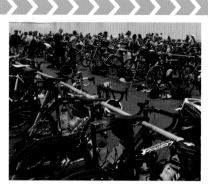

**1 PRE-RACE PREPARATION** Walk through the transition area to locate the "swim in" and look for markers that will help you identify where your bike is racked when you exit the water.

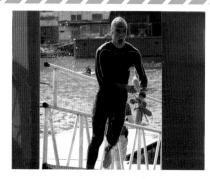

**2 EXIT THE WATER** As soon as you get out of the water, start running towards T1. You may feel slightly dizzy as blood rushes to your legs. If this happens, just relax and walk for a few metres.

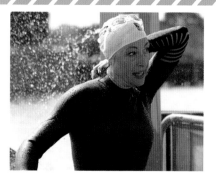

**3 GOGGLES ON YOUR HEAD** Put your goggles on your head to clear your vision and keep your hands free. Unzip your wetsuit as you move along: outside assistance is not allowed, so stay calm.

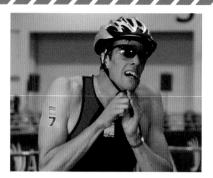

**7 HELMET ON, WETSUIT OFF** Put your helmet on as you stamp on your wetsuit to get it off. Your race belt/number can be worn under your wetsuit - or put it on now, along with your bike shoes (if they're not on to the pedals).

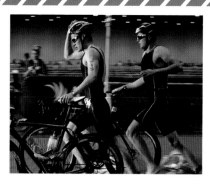

**8 GRAB YOUR BIKE AND RUN** Unrack your bike and start running to the "bike out" exit (riding your bike before reaching the mount line will lead to a time penalty). Hold the seat as you run with the bike.

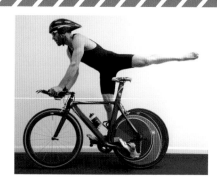

**9 MOUNT YOUR BIKE** Elite cyclists use a "flying mount" as the most efficient way to get going, but it takes practice. Novice triathletes may find it easier to "scoot on" (with one foot on a pedal) or stop the bike and swing a leg over.

## T1 SET-UP

Preparation will save time in transition. Place your kit on a towel next to your bike with separate sections for cycling and running gear. Have an extra water bottle to rinse dirt and grit off your feet after the swim. Go through your checklist to ensure you have everything before heading off to race.

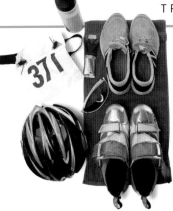

### CHECKLIST

- Bike shoes (on bike)
- Bike helmet
- Race belt
- Running shoes
- Water bottle (on bike)
- Nutrition
- Transition towel
- Elastic bands (for shoes on bike)
- Bike computer (calibrated)

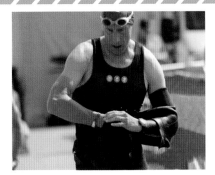

**4 PEEL OFF WETSUIT** Take off your wetsuit on the run to T1. Take your arms out first, then push the wetsuit down to your hips (keep the goggles and hat on your head so your hands are free).

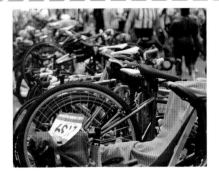

**5 LOCATE YOUR BIKE** Look for the markers to help you find your bike and run towards your transition spot. As you approach your bike, take off your hat and goggles.

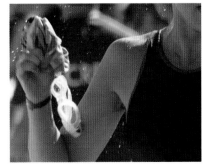

**6 AT YOUR BIKE** Throw your hat and goggles either into the basket provided or onto the floor next to your bike. Push your wetsuit as far down your legs as it will go.

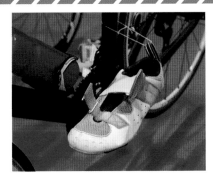

**10 GET PEDALLING** If your shoes are attached to the pedals, put your feet in them as you mount the bike. If you can't do this straight away, get up to "race pace" before you try again. Momentum is everything at this point.

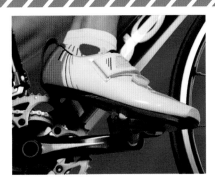

**11 MAINTAIN MOMENTUM** You will slow down as you put your foot in the shoe, so get back up to race pace before inserting the other. If there is a hill outside T1, make sure you get up it before putting your feet into the shoes.

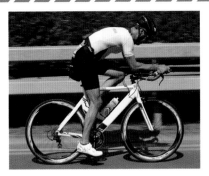

**12 HAVE FUN ON THE BIKE!** Remember that setting off too quickly in the excitement of getting on the bike could mean that you end up walking on the run. Keep focused on your race plan and adapt as necessary.

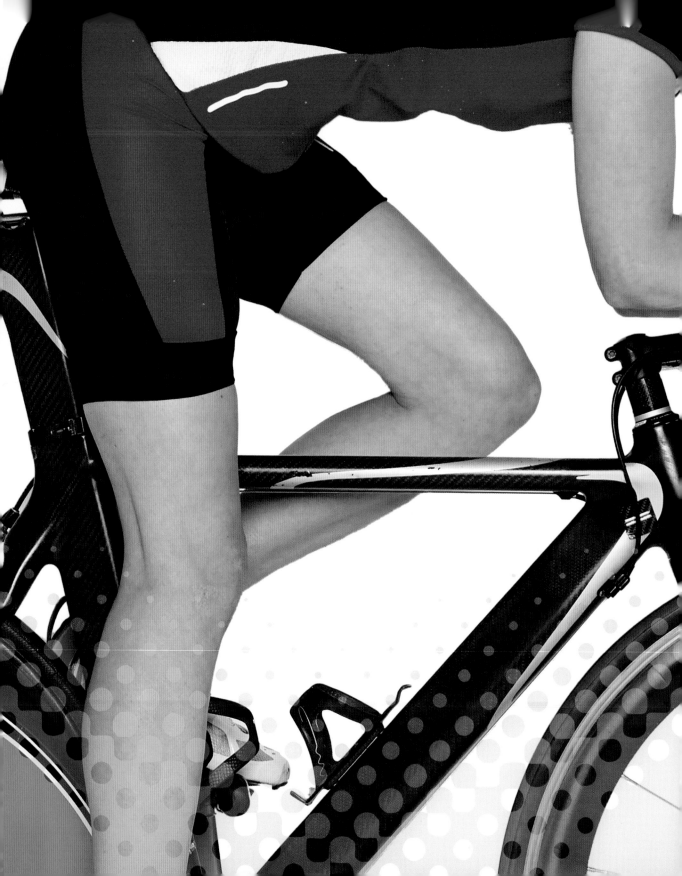

# THE
# CYCLING LAB

# THE BIKE

**For this stage** of the triathlon, it is all too easy to become obsessed by equipment. If you train hard, you can do your first triathlon on any kind of bike so long as it is roadworthy. The two main types of bike used in triathlons are the road bike and the time-trial, or tri, bike. The difference in performance can be significant, but there are arguments in favour of either option.

**❝ THINK AND TRY BEFORE YOU BUY:** EACH BIKE TYPE HAS **ADVANTAGES** IN PARTICULAR SETTINGS, AND **BUYING** THE WRONG BIKE IS AN EXPENSIVE MISTAKE. ❞

## ROAD BIKE

The road bike is what you will see in any regular age-group bike race, and is used by elite Olympic-distance athletes. For beginners, its proportions make for a more upright and comfortable ride, and better bike handling than a tri bike. It is ideally suited to normal road and group riding, as you ride with your head higher up and your hands closer to the brakes, giving you better vision and a quicker reaction time to road conditions, other cyclists, and traffic.

**» ROAD BIKES: WHAT KIT DO YOU NEED AS YOU IMPROVE?**

| PROGRESSION | NOVICE | IMPROVER | EXPERIENCED |
|---|---|---|---|
| FOOTWEAR | TRAINERS | TRAINERS OR STIFFER SHOES | BIKE SHOES AND CLEATS |
| PEDALS | FLAT | TOE CLIPS | CLIP-IN PEDALS |
| TRI-BARS | NONE | NONE | CLIP-ON AEROBARS |
| WHEELS FOR RACING | NORMAL | SLIGHT DEEP RIM | DEEPER RIMS |

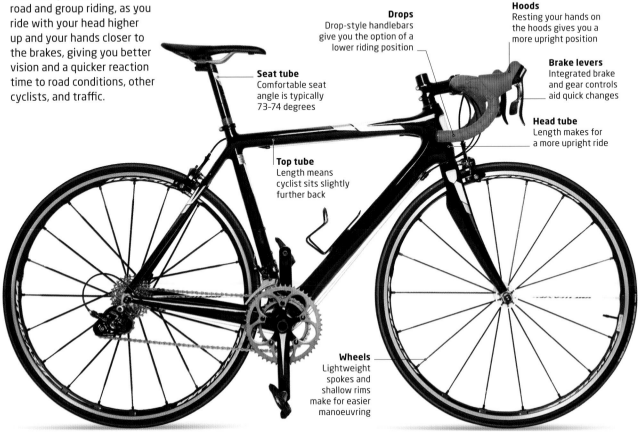

**Drops**
Drop-style handlebars give you the option of a lower riding position

**Hoods**
Resting your hands on the hoods gives you a more upright position

**Brake levers**
Integrated brake and gear controls aid quick changes

**Head tube**
Length makes for a more upright ride

**Seat tube**
Comfortable seat angle is typically 73-74 degrees

**Top tube**
Length means cyclist sits slightly further back

**Wheels**
Lightweight spokes and shallow rims make for easier manoeuvring

## COMPARE POSITIONS

Road bikes have a more relaxed geometry than tri bikes and can be more comfortable to ride at first. Tri bikes have a steeper seat angle, pushing the rider forwards and dropping their front end to optimize the aerodynamics of the rider and machine.

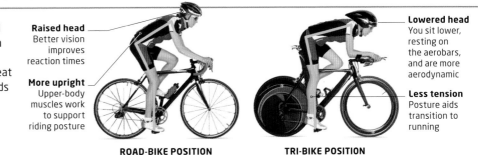

**Raised head**
Better vision improves reaction times

**More upright**
Upper-body muscles work to support riding posture

**ROAD-BIKE POSITION**

**Lowered head**
You sit lower, resting on the aerobars, and are more aerodynamic

**Less tension**
Posture aids transition to running

**TRI-BIKE POSITION**

## TRI BIKE

The tri bike, with its emphasis on aerodynamics, is designed for open roads and non-drafting races (see pp.52–53), and optimizes speed. It also aids running in the final leg of the triathlon – because you sit further forwards on the bike, your quads are more dominant as you power down on the pedals, which means your hamstrings will be less fatigued when you run.

**» TRI BIKES: WHAT KIT DO YOU NEED AS YOU IMPROVE?**

| PROGRESSION | NOVICE | IMPROVER | EXPERIENCED |
|---|---|---|---|
| HELMET | ROAD HELMET | AERO HELMET | AERO HELMET / VISOR |
| WHEELS | LIGHTER WHEELS OR DEEPER RIMS | TRI SPOKE REAR AND 404 FRONT | DISC REAR AND 808 FRONT |
| ADDITIONAL KIT | Q RINGS ON CHAIN'S CRANKSET | POWER METER | FINE TUNING OF BIKE FIT AND RIDING POSITION |

**Aero bars**
Resting on the aeros enhances comfort and aerodynamics

**Gears**
Controls located at the top of the aerobars allow quick changes

**Seat tube**
Typical seat angle of 76–78 degrees moves the cyclist forwards over the pedal

**Head tube**
Shorter head tube gives a more aerodynamic cycling position

**Top tube**
Shorter top tube so you sit forwards

**Wheels**
Deep front rim and rear disc cut air resistance and increase speed

# BIKE FIT

**Getting your bike** set up to fit you correctly will do wonders for your cycling. The key outcome from this five-stage beginner's bike fit is comfort, which will in turn increase power and efficiency. You need to understand the principles, but get your local specialist bike shop to help you with the fit.

## PROFESSIONAL ADVICE

The advice given here is for a standard road bike. A tri bike will require a different set of measurements to enhance aerodynamics and ensure maximum comfort, power, and efficiency. Whatever kind of bike you use, a specialist bike shop should be able to help.

### AERODYNAMICS

Aerodynamics only comes into play at speeds of more than 40kph (25mph). Elite cyclists aim for a slightly curved back, which creates a single, more streamlined curve from the aero helmet to the buttocks, reducing the drag that comes into play behind the rider.

**Reduced drag**
Smoother air flow creates less drag, the negative force holding you back

**Curved surface**
Air flows more readily over curved surfaces than flat ones

**Rear disc**
Many elite cyclists use a disc wheel to reduce drag at the rear

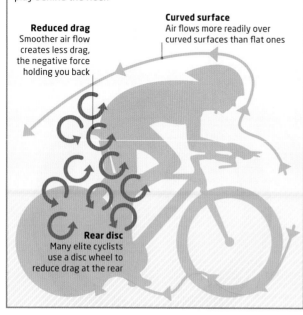

**1 TOP TUBE**
When deciding on a suitable bike, simply stand over the bike to test the height. The top tube should be around 2.5cm (1 inch) below your groin.

**2 SADDLE HEIGHT**
To get the correct saddle height, sit on the seat and put the ball of your foot on the pedal (wearing the shoes you will be riding in). When your foot is at 6 o'clock (the bottom of the pedal stroke) you should have a slight bend in the knee. If the saddle height is right, there should be no hip-rocking while you pedal.

## 4 REACH
Lean forwards with your hands on top of the bars on the hoods (around the brake housing). You should not be over-reaching or cramped up. Don't move your saddle back or forth; instead lengthen or shorten its stem to adjust.

**Elbow bend**
In Step 4, your elbow should have a natural bend – don't over-reach

## 5 GRIP
The space between the brake levers and the handlebar drops needs to allow for comfortable braking. Women with smaller hands may need to adjust the set-up.

2.5cm (1 inch)

## 3 POWER POSITION
To find the correct seat position, bring your feet level at 3 and 9 o'clock, then:
- Align your front knee between the second and third toe
- Take a piece of string with a small weight attached
- Place the non-weighted end against the little bump under your knee and let the weight drop down
- The weight needs to be over the centre of the pedal, where the maximum force will be generated

**The right height**
Position the pedal down at 6 o'clock for Step 2

## AEROBARS FIT
If attaching aerobars to a road bike, try to find a balance between aerodynamics and comfort. In elite racing, aerobars must not extend beyond the brake hoods.

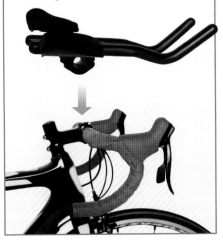

## CLEAT FIT
There will usually be some float (movement between cleat and pedal), so have your feet pointing forwards at all times. The knuckle of your big toe needs to align with the centre of the pedal, as this is where the maximum force will come through.

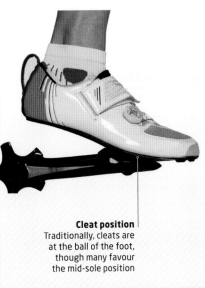

**Cleat position**
Traditionally, cleats are at the ball of the foot, though many favour the mid-sole position

# ANATOMY OF A CYCLIST

**In cycling, unlike swimming,** it is the lower part of the body that provides power and forward motion. Each stroke or rotation of the pedal consists of a power and momentum phase. Understanding how your legs work through these phases helps you to generate maximum power.

## KEY »

The main muscles used in cycling are the quadriceps, gluteals, hip flexors, hamstrings, and calf muscles. The quads, gluteals, and calves do most of the work in the power phase; the other muscles help you to smooth your pedalling action (see pp.44–45).

- QUADRICEPS
- GLUTEALS
- HIP FLEXORS
- HAMSTRINGS
- GASTROCNEMIUS
- SOLEUS
- TIBIALIS ANTERIOR

## POWER

The leg powers down from the top of the stroke. The quads do most of the work at the start of the stroke, then the gluteals and calf muscles take over towards the bottom as you push the pedal through the bottom of the stroke. Learning to utilize the full range of muscles will help you avoid fatigue and leave you with enough energy for the run.

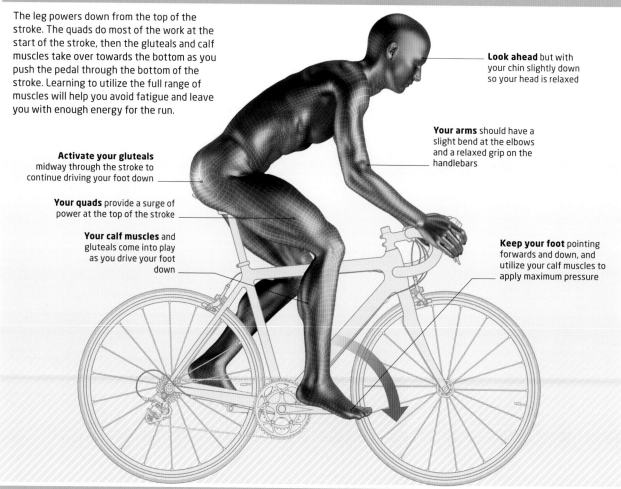

**Activate your gluteals** midway through the stroke to continue driving your foot down

**Your quads** provide a surge of power at the top of the stroke

**Your calf muscles** and gluteals come into play as you drive your foot down

**Look ahead** but with your chin slightly down so your head is relaxed

**Your arms** should have a slight bend at the elbows and a relaxed grip on the handlebars

**Keep your foot** pointing forwards and down, and utilize your calf muscles to apply maximum pressure

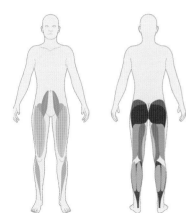

# THE KINETIC CHAIN

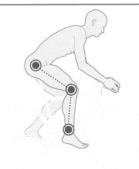

The kinetic chain is made up of your muscles, tendons, ligaments, joints, fascia, and neural system working as one. Each component is dependent on the next. With cycling, the kinetic chain that runs from the hips to the feet is key. As you press down through the power phase, any weak link – such as a sore knee – will affect your pedalling and limit your power production. Good cycling techique is key to avoiding those weaknesses.

## MOMENTUM

The second phase of the cycling stroke is momentum. Your leg is now resting while the majority of the work is being done by the other leg in its power phase. To maintain your momentum, lift the foot of your resting leg out of the way and let the pedal push you back into the power phase.

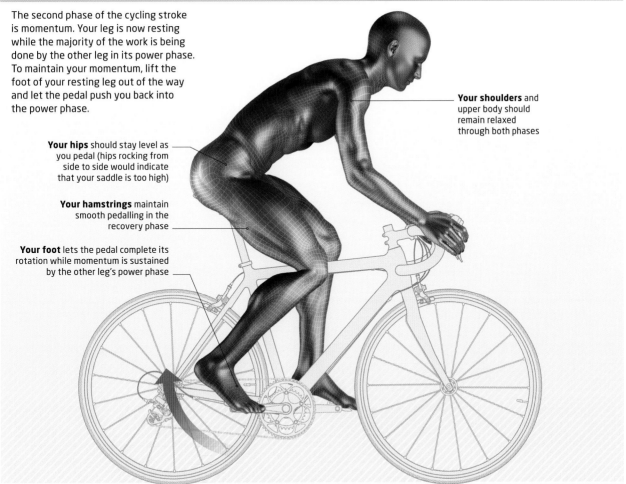

**Your shoulders** and upper body should remain relaxed through both phases

**Your hips** should stay level as you pedal (hips rocking from side to side would indicate that your saddle is too high)

**Your hamstrings** maintain smooth pedalling in the recovery phase

**Your foot** lets the pedal complete its rotation while momentum is sustained by the other leg's power phase

# EFFICIENT CYCLING

**The best way to think** of efficient cycling is to imagine making smooth, fluid strokes around the whole revolution. As well as studying the technique involved, becoming efficient requires hours of practice on the bike. When good technique becomes ingrained, it will feel completely natural.

## PEDAL STROKE PHASES

The power and momentum phases described on pp.42-43 can be further broken down into four pedal stroke phases. The downstroke is where most of the power is concentrated, but it is the complete flowing motion that is important for efficiency.

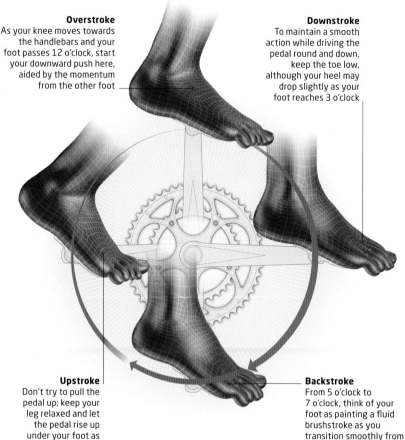

**Overstroke**
As your knee moves towards the handlebars and your foot passes 12 o'clock, start your downward push here, aided by the momentum from the other foot

**Downstroke**
To maintain a smooth action while driving the pedal round and down, keep the toe low, although your heel may drop slightly as your foot reaches 3 o'clock

**Upstroke**
Don't try to pull the pedal up; keep your leg relaxed and let the pedal rise up under your foot as the opposite foot powers down

**Backstroke**
From 5 o'clock to 7 o'clock, think of your foot as painting a fluid brushstroke as you transition smoothly from your power phase into the momentum phase.

## ALIGNMENT

When you pedal efficiently, your legs pump up and down like pistons, with little or no sideways movement at the knee, which should remain aligned over your big toe. Your hips should be square (level) and still; rocking from side to side indicates that your seat is too high, which will prevent you driving your foot down correctly during the power phase (see p.42). Keep your shoulders relaxed, your chin slightly down, and your arms slightly bent with a relaxed grip on the bars.

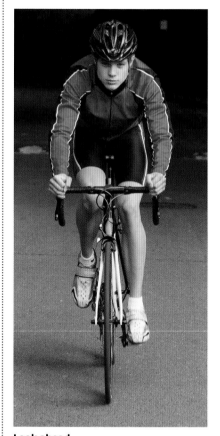

**Look ahead**
Efficient cycling should look relaxed, showing no unnecessary movement. The less energy you use while cycling, the more you will have left for the run.

## FINDING THE RIGHT CADENCE

Cadence refers to pedalling speed, measured in revolutions per minute (rpm). Many triathletes favour high cadences, in the 90-100rpm range, although some go far lower. It is easier to pedal in a lower gear, but you need a very high cadence to maintain your pace. A higher gear lets you do that at a lower cadence, but requires more power.

- If you are new to cycling, start by learning to spin smooth revolutions at 90-100rpm (see pp.46-47), then move to higher gears at 55-75rpm and see what you prefer.

- Experiment with riding at different cadences to see how they make your legs feel once you transition from bike to run (see pp.56-57).

- When you have found the best cadence for you, experiment with gearing so you can maintain your cadence on different courses (see pp.52-53).

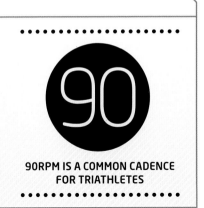

**90RPM IS A COMMON CADENCE FOR TRIATHLETES**

# CORNERING

Successful cornering is about maintaining speed through the corner. The leaning method shown here works well for smooth corners at high speeds. For lower speeds, very sharp corners, or wet road conditions, you will also need to steer.

**Approach**

**Apex**

**Exit**

**Watch your space**
When riding on a road, consider the space you take up; adjust your cornering line to accommodate other road users.

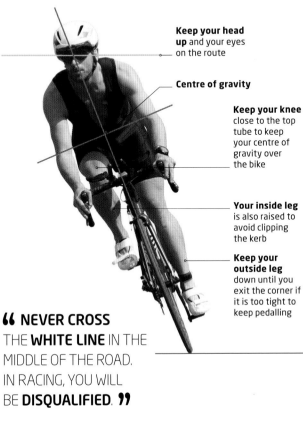

**Keep your head up** and your eyes on the route

**Centre of gravity**

**Keep your knee** close to the top tube to keep your centre of gravity over the bike

**Your inside leg** is also raised to avoid clipping the kerb

**Keep your outside leg** down until you exit the corner if it is too tight to keep pedalling

**❝ NEVER CROSS** THE **WHITE LINE** IN THE MIDDLE OF THE ROAD. IN RACING, YOU WILL BE **DISQUALIFIED. ❞**

### 1 Approach
As you approach a corner or roundabout, keep your head up and try to look through the bend and beyond. Slow down if necessary and select the gear you will need for coming out of the corner - avoid the risk of braking too hard and the distraction of changing gear and losing momentum while you corner.

### 2 Entry
Enter the corner at a speed you are comfortable with. Keep looking through and beyond the corner, and try to identify the apex (the straightest/fastest line through the corner). You may need to adjust this line to avoid potholes or others on the road.

### 3 Through the corner
For a right turn, for example, ensure that your outside (left) foot is down at 6 o'clock with your weight pressing through it to steady the bike. Your inside (right) foot will be up at 12 o'clock. Your weight is still centred over your bike. Let the bike lean into the corner.

### 4 Exit
Having come through the corner, keep this head-up riding going as you straighten the bike and get back up to speed. As you have already selected the right gear for exiting the corner, you can now get out of your seat and pedal using your bodyweight to help you accelerate back up to your race pace.

# CYCLING DRILLS

**The best way** to become a better cyclist is to go out and ride for a long time as often as possible. However, using your bike on an indoor training turbo or on rollers at the gym will also enhance your skills. Use a cadence counter to check your rpm.

## 01 SINGLE-LEG TURBO

This drill will smooth your pedalling action and help to eliminate any clunking sounds in your revolutions. Start in an easy gear.

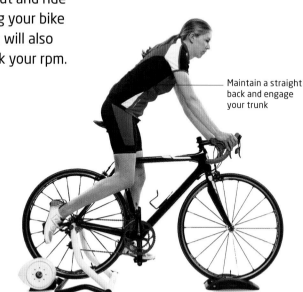

Maintain a straight back and engage your trunk

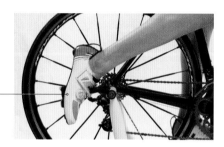

Place the non-working leg on the back of the turbo, away from the wheel

1 Once you are set up with your bike on the turbo, warm up with an easy spin, pedalling with both legs for 5-10 minutes. Then unclip your right foot and rest it on the back of the turbo.

2 Pedal with your left leg at 90-95rpm for 30 seconds, keeping your action smooth. If you can hear a clunking sound, try lifting your knee over the top of the revolution. Then pedal using both legs for 30 seconds, before switching to the other side for 30 seconds. Repeat 10 times to complete the set.

## 02 NO-CHAIN TURBO

Removing the chain will help you work on the top part of the revolution, which will increase the smoothness of your pedalling.

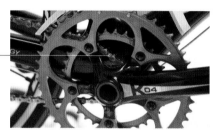

Rest the chain on the inside of the chainring

1 Carefully remove the chain from the chainring. Once on the turbo, unclip your right foot and place it on the back of the turbo. Keep the cadence lower on this drill, at about 55-60rpm.

2 Pedal at about 55-60rpm until your leg tires; to begin with, this will be after about 20-40 seconds. Then switch to the other side and do the same repetitions as for the Single-leg drill.

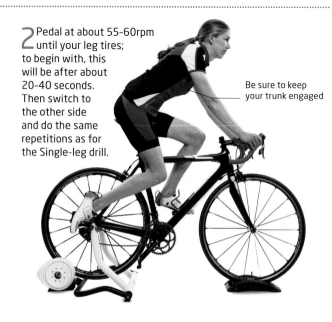

Be sure to keep your trunk engaged

# 03 **SPIN-UPS** TURBO

Once you've mastered the single-leg drills, get going with both legs at once. Spin-ups are simple drills that help smooth out your pedalling action and develop your cycling neural pathways.

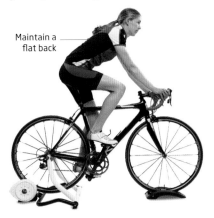

Maintain a flat back

**Pedal in a medium gear** at a moderate speed to warm your legs up. Gradually increase to 95rpm, and maintain this cadence for one minute. Move up to 100rpm, 105rpm, 110rpm, 115rpm, and 120rpm, staying at each cadence for one minute. Keep your pedalling smooth, and if you encounter bouncing at a high cadence, try to relax your quads a little. Once you have completed one set, have an easy 5-minute spin and then go back down:
120 – 115 – 110 – 105 – 100 – 95rpm.

## HYPER CADENCE

Hyper cadence drills help train you to spin efficiently at very high cadences. They may be performed on a turbo trainer or on rollers. If using rollers, make sure that you are stable first – the drill will accentuate bouncing or imbalance in your cycling. Pedal at the cadences below for one minute each, or as fast as you can:

**105 - 110 - 115 - 120 - 125 - 130rpm**

Have a 5-minute spin at the end, then try to come back down the revolutions.

# 04 **ROLLERS** DRILL

Rollers are another great option for honing your skills, but getting started can be a challenge, so take frequent breaks. Position the rollers on a flat surface in between a wall and a mat, or in a doorway where you can lean against the frame – or ask a friend to hold the bike frame for you.

## PROGRESSION

**Once you can maintain stability**, try cycling with only one hand on the handlebars. Move onto cycling with no hands, and then onto the single-leg and spin-up drills with hands.

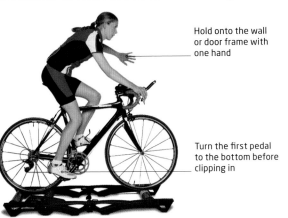

Hold onto the wall or door frame with one hand

Turn the first pedal to the bottom before clipping in

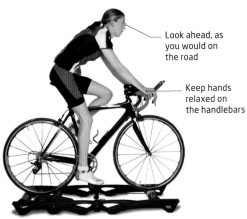

Look ahead, as you would on the road

Keep hands relaxed on the handlebars

1 Position the bicycle upright on the rollers, ensuring that it is in an easy gear. Clip your foot into the first pedal, hold onto the wall or door frame, and pull yourself over into the saddle, tilting the bicycle for balance. Clip in your other foot.

2 Once comfortable, place your stabilizing hand on the handlebars. Start to pedal and get up to a high cadence (90-95rpm), hold this for about 60 seconds, and then take a break. Gradually build up the time you can ride.

# BIKE SESSIONS

**Choose your training sessions** according to the time of year and your performance goals. Five levels of training intensity are shown below. Most of your sessions should be at Levels 1 and 2, with a smaller proportion of higher-level sessions to enhance aspects of your race performance. Working on technical elements will help you achieve improved economy, while working on extending your physical capabilities will bring increases in speed and power - leading to a faster overall time for the bike section in the triathlon, and fresher legs for the run.

## CYCLING WARM-UP

For a relaxed ride at Level 1 or 2, warm up by riding steadily for 10-20 minutes and build the pace up slowly. Before Level 3-5 sessions, you need to carry out a thorough warm-up:

- 5 minutes - easy spin (low gear)
- 5 minutes - build to race pace effort
- 5 x 15 seconds at 95 per cent effort sprinting in a big gear (out of your seat), with 45 seconds easy spin in between
- 5-10 minutes - easy spin

# TRAINING LEVELS 1-5

## 1 EASY

This session is about time in the saddle and improving your fat utilization (see pp.90-91) over a long steady distance (LSD).

**TARGET:** 56-70 per cent of functional threshold power (FTP, which is the maximum power you can sustain for 1 hour: see pp.50-51), or 50-60 per cent of your maximum heart rate (HR max), at a comfortable cadence for you.

**MAIN SET:** Choose one of the following options:
- 90 minutes plus, OR
- Ride for up to 6 hours; build up to this

**RECOVERY:** Hot shower or bath.

**PROGRESSION:** Start with a steady cycle for 90 minutes. Increase distance by 10 per cent every ride, until you reach your goal, e.g. 100km (65 miles).

**BENEFITS:** Builds endurance; the key part is the mental endurance of the long steady ride, along with the physical benefits described above.

## 2 TEMPO

As with swimming, this level is about bringing a little more rhythm to your ride, at or around your race cadence. It can also be used for force work - riding up a hill with a low cadence (rpm) and a harder gear.

**TARGET:** 68-78 per cent of FTP, or 60-70 per cent HR max.

**MAIN SET:** Choose one of these sets:
- 6 x 5 minutes at 55 rpm with 5-minute easy spin between, OR
- 3 x 10 minutes at 65 rpm with 8-minute easy spin between, OR
- 1 x 20 minutes at 75 rpm with 10-minute easy spin between

**RECOVERY:** A few minutes of spinning (95-105 rpm), or extended spinning time to loosen the legs.

**PROGRESSION:** Aim to increase resistance or make repetitions longer.

**BENEFITS:** Increased cycling power and smooth pedalling action.

## 3 THRESHOLD

This is race-pace work at the personal race cadence that feels most efficient and can be sustained.

**TARGET:** 95-100 per cent of FTP, or 70-85 per cent HR max.

**MAIN SET:** Choose one of these sets:
- 4 x 10 minutes cycling at your race cadence (e.g. 90-100 rpm), with 5 minutes recovery between sets, OR
- 2 x 20 minutes at 90-100 rpm, 10 minutes recovery between sets, OR
- Race distance: warm up, then either 30 minutes/20km or 60 minutes/40km time trial (racing alone against the clock)

**RECOVERY:** Take about half of the time in the repetition to cool down.

**PROGRESSION:** Reduce recovery times or increase duration of each set.

**BENEFITS:** Develops your race pacing and increases your pain tolerance.

## SAMPLE SESSION

This sample session from Level 2 shows you how to structure a session around your main set. The levels below offer a choice of sets. Select one, increasing by 10 per cent every session until you can complete any of the sets listed. Focus on key areas to improve and aim to complete three different bike sessions per week.

*For a sample foundation programme of weekly sessions, see pp.122-123.*

| L2 SESSION | SAMPLE ACTIVITY |
|---|---|
| WARM-UP | Steady pace ride in easy gear for 10-20 minutes: increases your heart rate, focuses the mind |
| PRE-MAIN DRILL SET | Harder gear, increase cadence: 30 seconds left leg, 30 seconds right x 10 (outdoors or on turbo) |
| MAIN SET | e.g. 6 x 5 minutes at 55 rpm with 5-minute spin between: moderate increase in effort, in a higher gear |
| COOL-DOWN | Easy 5-minute ride: winds your body down slowly after a tempo ride, reducing risk of injury |

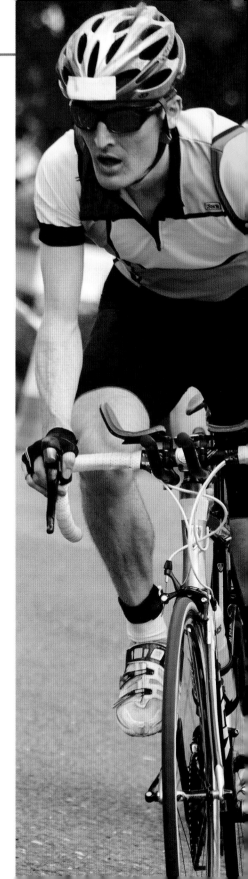

## 4 vVO2 MAX

An intense session to raise your vVO2 max (speed at which you reach maximal oxygen consumption).

**TARGET:** 100-103 per cent of FTP, or 85-96 per cent of HR max.

**MAIN SET:** Choose one of these sets:
- 3 x 6 minutes cycling at 100 per cent effort In a hard gear and around race cadence, with 6 minutes recovery between sets in lower gear, OR
- Hill: up a hill with a gradient of 6-12 per cent for 1-3 minutes; drop just below threshold to dissipate lactate for 3-6 minutes

**RECOVERY:** Continue easy pedalling for the same time as the repetition.

**PROGRESSION:** Work harder as you get fitter, or reduce the recovery time.

**BENEFITS:** Increases your vVO2 max and also speeds up recovery from short sprints or climbs by dissipating lactate (see p.160) from hard-working muscles.

## 5 MAXIMAL

These are intense sessions at 100 per cent of your HR max.

**TARGET:** 103-180 per cent of FTP, or 96-100 per cent of HR max.

**MAIN SET:**
It is essential that you do a thorough warm-up first (see Cycling warm-up, top left), then work through these in turn:
- 15-20 x 30-second sprints
- 6 x 3 minutes at threshold, then out of the seat and sprint for 40 seconds
- Tempo uphill, then out of the seat and sprint for 10 seconds
Allow full recovery between each.

**RECOVERY:** You will need 48 hours before another intense session.

**PROGRESSION:** Increase resistance or repetitions.

**BENEFITS:** Improved economy and power, as well as increased fast-twitch muscle recruitment (see p.160).

For more details on how Levels 1-5 target physiology and fitness, see pp.160-161.

# ASSESSING YOUR BIKE FITNESS

**Cycling is affected** by numerous factors – from weather to road surfaces – all of which may mean you use up more energy than planned, leaving you short for the last leg. And so it is crucial to assess your bike fitness. Visit your doctor for a check-up and take the general fitness tests on pp.28–29 before you begin.

### Q WHAT ARE THE FACTORS THAT CAN VARY?

**A** Cycling is basically pedalling against resistance, but if you are training outdoors, that resistance can be constantly changing. Small inclines, rougher or smoother surfaces, gusts of wind, and "false flats" (sections of road that look flat but aren't really) will all affect your Rate of Perceived Exertion (RPE, see p.29) and may give you a false impression of how you're doing.

### Q SO HOW CAN I MONITOR MY WORK RATE?

**A** One solution is to use a power meter – an electrical gauge attached to the bike's crank for measuring the turning force (torque) you apply to the pedals. It gives you real-time effort levels in power units called watts (W). Its advantage over a heart rate (HR) monitor is that it doesn't have a time-lag. For example, on a false flat, your HR may have gone up 20 beats per minute but it may be a few minutes before this registers on your HR monitor.

Alternatively, schedule a regular session in an indoor gym and use one of the cycling machines there to measure your power output.

### Q WILL SPEED MATTER DURING MY RIDE?

**A** In triathlon cycling, power output is far more important than speed. This is because if your race pace is, say, 30kph (19mph) but you are riding into a headwind of 10kph (6mph), you will have to slow down or risk consuming so much energy that you run the final leg at less than your optimal speed, or even end up walking it.

### Q WHERE SHOULD I DO MY BIKE FITNESS TESTS?

**A** You need to find a course where you won't be held up by traffic or obstacles. Make sure it is as flat as possible: downhill slopes allow you to freewheel, which won't test you. Choose a quiet, distraction-free route to allow for maximum concentration. Alternatively, use a gym bike that records power. Repeat each test on these pages every 8–12 weeks.

---

## TAKE THE FTP TEST

Functional Threshold Power (FTP) is the average power you can sustain for an hour. The higher your FTP, the stronger you are. Because cycling is all about endurance in changing circumstances, the FTP is the best measure of your fitness. However, it is difficult to measure yourself over a full hour, so a 20-minute session is the standard indicator in biking.

### WHAT TO DO

1 **Warm-up** Do the cycle warm-up before you begin the test (see p.52).

2 **Calibrate** Whether you have a power meter on your bike or are using a bike in a gym, make sure that you reset the device after your warm up to ensure that you collect only the data for the time trial (TT).

3 **Cycle 20 minutes** Time trialling is all about hitting and holding a sustainable pace, and your warm-up will enable you to get up to your TT pace straight away. Keep up this pace, and if you have gone out at the right level you may have a little energy left at the end to drive the pace harder for around 20–30 seconds. Have a friend there to make sure you are okay after the test.

4 **Cool down** Ask your friend to record the data you have just produced, as you will be exhausted and probably in no fit state to do much apart from recover. If you are on your own, make sure that you press "SAVE" on your device.

### WHAT TO RECORD

So long as you press "SAVE" on your device, most of the data below will be saved automatically. But check this with a test run prior to the real thing.

• **Average power output** The power output from your meter or gym bike will be given in watts (W).

## DO A 16KM (10-MILE) TIME TRIAL

The test is simple: simply ride your bike as fast as you can for 16km (10 miles). It is less accurate than an FTP test, because your ride time is likely to be influenced by variables such as weather. But if you can ride the same course each time on days with similar conditions, it can be a great way to track your progress.

**WHAT TO RECORD**
• Time taken to ride 16km (10 miles)
• Average and maximum heart rate
• Average cadence, average speed

**HOW DO YOU RATE?**
The best cyclists can finish in under 20 minutes. Most beginners will take more than 30 minutes.

## ASSESS YOUR POWER-TO-WEIGHT RATIO (PWR)

Use a gym bike or a power meter to calculate the effect of your body mass on your cycling (it takes more power to move a heavier body). The higher your power-to-weight ratio, the better you will perform, especially on inclines and hills.

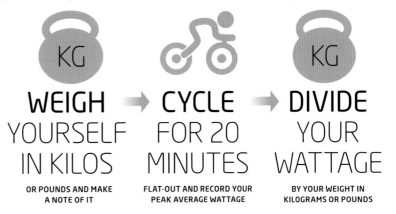

**WEIGH YOURSELF IN KILOS**
OR POUNDS AND MAKE A NOTE OF IT

**CYCLE FOR 20 MINUTES**
FLAT-OUT AND RECORD YOUR PEAK AVERAGE WATTAGE

**DIVIDE YOUR WATTAGE**
BY YOUR WEIGHT IN KILOGRAMS OR POUNDS

**For example,** if you weigh 75kg (165lb) and can keep up 423 watts for 20 minutes, the figure will be 423 divided by 75, or 6.64W/kg (2.56W/lb). Such a high PWR would rank you as "exceptional/domestic pro". Your own PWR results are likely to be more modest, especially when just starting out.

• **Normalized power (NP)** Riding a bike is not smooth, so the NP function on a power meter or gym bike effectively calculates the average power produced during your ride.

• **Average cadence** Cadence is the number of pedal revolutions per minute, and it is a useful objective measurement (see pp.44–45). A gym bike should measure it automatically. During your training you will get a feel for what cadence suits your riding type; however, it is still interesting to record this data during a TT as this will normally become your race cadence.

• **Average speed** Although speed is a true measure in cycling, you should record the conditions (if you are riding outdoors) and TT in similar conditions the next time you take the FTP test. You should see your speed increasing as your fitness improves.

• **Average heart rate (HR)** This will be about the same each time you test yourself, but you will see improvements in the other parameters you are measuring. You won't get to a maximum HR, but you will see a sub-max HR for your TT pace.

### FINDING YOUR FTP

To calculate your FTP score, take the average power figure recorded by your meter or the gym exercise bike for the 20-minute test. Then multiply that figure by 0.95. So if your average output was 300W, your FTP will be: 300 x 0.95 = 285W.

### HOW DO YOU RATE?

Compare your current FTP score with the world of cycling in charts online. Use your profiling tools and goal setting to improve your cycling.

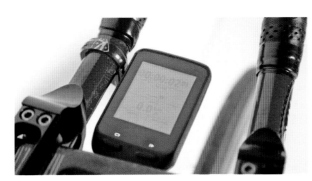

The power meter's screen attaches to the bike's handlebars or handlebar stem. This meter tells you which training levels (see pp.48–49) you should be in during each part of the FTP test.

# ON THE ROAD

**Road cycling, or live riding,** helps you to familiarize yourself with how to handle your bike in different conditions all through the year. Riding on the open road is very different from riding on indoor trainers. Whether you are riding in a group or alone, remember to be safe and be seen; know the rules of the road as they apply to cyclists.

**IN THE PACK**

- When riding in a group, familiarize yourself with the hand signals to indicate stopping, slowing, parked cars, and potholes
- Don't rely on others - always carry what you need
- Keep aligned with the wheels of the rider in front and beside you
- Be courteous to all other road users

## YOUR ROUTE TO SUCCESS

### BE SELF-SUFFICIENT

Regardless of whether you are riding in a group or on your own, you should always carry certain items with you:

- Puncture repair kit (2 inner tubes, tyre levers, small hand pump or air canister)
- Fluid (in bottle carrier cages on your bike)
- Mobile phone (in a waterproof cover)
- Money / Bank card
- Nutrition
- Rain jacket (even if the sun is out)
- Sunglasses (clear or tinted)

Distribute items between the pockets on the back of your cycling jacket, with only your rain jacket in the central pocket - nothing hard - as it will help protect the base of your spine in the event of an accident. To ensure you stay visible, wear bright clothing at all times.

### RIDING IN GOOD WEATHER

By far the busiest time on the roads is when the sun is out and the weather is good. However, this is also when you need to remain vigilant and be sensible about your road riding - stay hydrated, wear sunscreen on exposed parts of your body, and take lights and a rain jacket in case the conditions change. If it does turn wet, make sure your tyre pressure is a little lower (around 80-90psi) so your bike grips the road. Use your rear brake more than the front one in the rain so you stay in control.

### RIDING IN BAD WEATHER

Live riding can be undertaken all year round, but when conditions are dangerous or unpredictable (whether it's ice, snow, hailstorms, thunderstorms, or gale-force winds), your time will be much better spent practising indoors on a turbo trainer or rollers (see pp.46-47). Mountain biking is also a good alternative when bad weather rules out road cycling, and can enhance your general bike-handling skills.

# USING THE CORRECT GEARS

For road bikes, a typical gear combination has two chainrings at the front (with 53 and 39 "teeth" respectively) and 11 cogs on the rear cassette (with 11 to 28 teeth). You can choose to tailor your combinations. An easier (lighter) combination is a small chainring and larger rear cog - this can aid ascents as it helps you to retain a higher cadence (see p.45). A harder (heavier) combination is a large chainring and smaller rear cog, which can accelerate your pace during descents or over flat stretches.

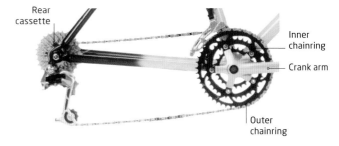

Rear cassette

Inner chainring

Crank arm

Outer chainring

## DRAFTING

Drafting is where you take your pace from a rider in front of you. By cycling in their slipstream, you are protected from the wind and are able to save energy while maintaining a steady speed. Elite triathletes do this in sprint and Olympic distance racing, and it is common practice during group training rides.

However, drafting is illegal in most age-group triathlon races, as well as for all athletes in half and full Ironman races. Competitors are only allowed to enter the draft zone of another athlete when passing them, and must keep going until they have overtaken them. All races have clear guidelines on this.

## PACING

Bike sessions (see pp.48-49) will help you understand your fitness levels, and what "race pace" means to you. As pacing during the bike section of a triathlon is key to optimum run performance, it is vital that you understand bike pacing. Start by finding your rate of perceived exertion (RPE), or the intensity of your exercise; one way of measuring this is with a heart-rate monitor (see p.29). The best option on the bike, though, is to use a power meter to find out how hard you are actually working, and to understand your functional threshold power, or FTP (see p.48).

## CHANGING GEAR

Gears make your cycling more efficient. Consider your cadence (see p.45) and experiment with different gears on climbs, descents, and on the flat. The correct cadence is specific to the rider, so when approaching an uphill or descent select a gear that is right for you. That gear selection must result in a similar torque (the amount of force needed to make the pedals rotate), RPE, heart rate, and power as on the flat, to enable you to conserve energy for the run. A gear that is too easy will result in a high cadence; too hard and you will build lactate and pedal inefficiently.

# WHAT TO WEAR

**When going out on your bike,** you need to wear appropriate cycling clothing. Make sure you take an essential repair kit with you and be prepared for variable weather conditions. All helmets worn in triathlons need to meet official safety standards, so make sure you buy one with the appropriate safety mark. Your local cycle shop will be able to advise you.

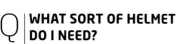

**40** KPH

AERODYNAMICS IS NOT AN ISSUE UNTIL YOU CYCLE AT 40KPH (25MPH) OR MORE

---

**Q WHAT SORT OF HELMET DO I NEED?**

**A** Choose a helmet that is comfortable and fits well. "Aero" helmets are designed to reduce wind resistance, but they have less ventilation – not so good over a long distance in the heat – and they are expensive. If you are a beginner, start with a standard road helmet. Aerodynamics will not be a significant factor until you can ride at around 40kph (25mph).

**Q WHICH TYPE OF SHOES DO I NEED?**

**A** The key is a good fit; cycling shoes need to be snug so they don't cause black toe nails (bleeding under the nail caused by pressure). If you are new to cycling, it is best to start with normal pedals that have either straps or toe clips. Once you are comfortable with these, you can progress to cleats and clip-in pedals (see box, opposite). Cleats produce a more efficient pedalling action (see p.44) and are safer than toe clips and straps as they

have a built-in safety mechanism that releases the foot from the pedal in a crash.

**Q WHAT SHOULD I WEAR IN COLD WEATHER?**

**A** In cool autumn weather, you may want to wear some arm- and knee-warmers, and possibly a gilet (a waistcoat-style top) to protect from the chill. In colder weather, thermal jackets, tights, booties, ear-warmers, and gloves will all help. You may also want to use heat pads in your shoes and gloves. Make sure that your tights or shorts have a good chamois pad in the seat to stop you getting saddle-sore. Some athletes prefer cycling tights with bibs (straps over the shoulders) as they stay in place better than shorts. In wet weather, wear a good rain jacket and waterproof booties.

**Q WHAT SHOULD I WEAR IN WARM WEATHER?**

**A** Warm weather does not present as many problems as the cold. A pair of cycling shorts and a short-sleeved cycling top

will keep you cool in summer. Even in warm weather it is a good idea to wear a pair of track mits (fingerless gloves) that have padding over the ulnar nerve as they will protect your hands if you fall. Sunglasses are essential in bright sunshine – they will not only protect your eyes from glare, but also from dust, stones, and other road debris.

**Q WHAT ELSE DO I NEED?**

**A** Whether you are riding alone or with companions, you should always be equipped with the correct kit to deal with emergencies. Cycling tops should have three pockets at the back to carry your equipment: put the waterproof in the middle pocket over the spine for extra padding. Avoid putting anything hard in the pockets, such as the pump, in case of accidents. You will need a good stock of high-factor sunscreen and chamois cream: this makes the pad in your shorts more hygienic and reduces the chances of infected saddle sores (see p.154).

# CYCLING CLOTHES

Cycling gear should be comfortable, practical, and safe. Tailor your clothes to the weather conditions and make sure you are well protected and streamlined.

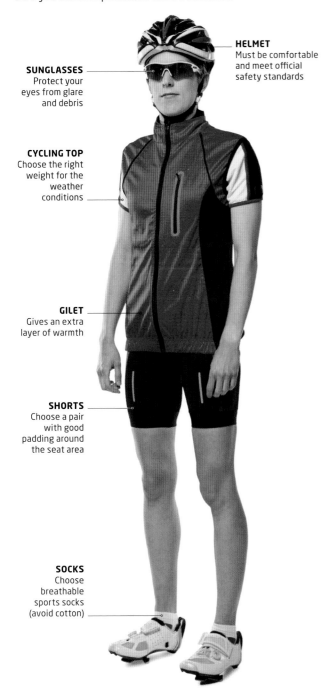

**SUNGLASSES**
Protect your eyes from glare and debris

**HELMET**
Must be comfortable and meet official safety standards

**CYCLING TOP**
Choose the right weight for the weather conditions

**GILET**
Gives an extra layer of warmth

**SHORTS**
Choose a pair with good padding around the seat area

**SOCKS**
Choose breathable sports socks (avoid cotton)

## HIGH-TECH CLOTHING

Worn close to the skin, high-tech fabrics are specially designed to pull, or "wick", moisture away from the skin's surface - the moisture from perspiration passes through to the outer side of the fabric, then evaporates. In contrast, clothing made from cotton retains sweat and can make you feel cold and clammy. Choose clothes that are lightweight, quick-drying, and close-fitting to allow freedom of movement on the bike. If the weather's cold, wear two or more layers to keep warm.

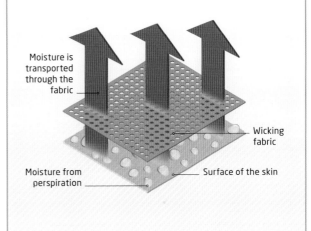

Moisture is transported through the fabric

Wicking fabric

Moisture from perspiration

Surface of the skin

## CLEATS

Considered safer and more efficient than toe clips and straps, cleats also provide a degree of "float" (movement between the cleat and pedal). This allows you to control the direction in which your toes point. For optimum pedalling, your toes should point forwards and the knuckle of your big toe should align with the centre of the pedal. If you are new to cleats and clip-in pedals, ask your local cycling shop for advice on fitting.

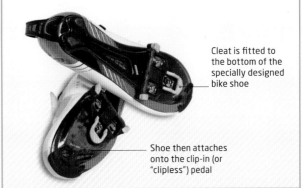

Cleat is fitted to the bottom of the specially designed bike shoe

Shoe then attaches onto the clip-in (or "clipless") pedal

# TRANSITION TWO (T2)

**When you change** from the bike leg to the run, you need to prepare for the only weight-bearing discipline of the race. Practising T2 and doing a few bike-to-run "brick" sessions during your training will really help with this section of the race.

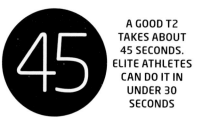

**45** A GOOD T2 TAKES ABOUT 45 SECONDS. ELITE ATHLETES CAN DO IT IN UNDER 30 SECONDS

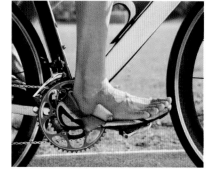

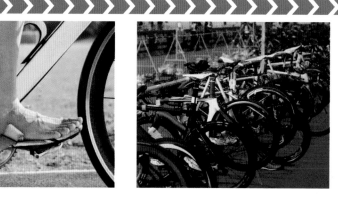

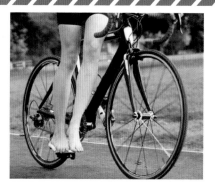

1 **SHOES OFF** Around 400m from the dismount line, take your feet out of your shoes and pedal with your feet on top of the shoes. Shift into an easier gear to get your legs ready for the run.

2 **PICTURE YOUR TRANSITION AREA** Visualize where your transition area is located. Remember landmarks and start to focus on getting there swiftly through the other athletes and bikes.

3 **GET OFF YOUR BIKE** Before the dismount line, stand on one pedal and swing your other leg round to join it. Touch down just before the line, as going over the line will result in time penalties.

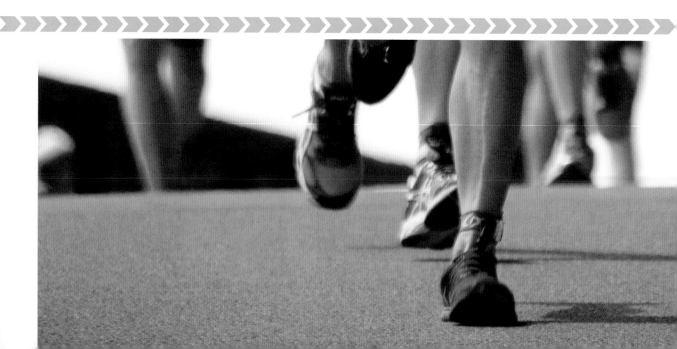

## T2 SET-UP

A smooth and efficient transition can save time and will set you up for the next leg of your race. Practice is key: don't allow adrenaline or haste to take over. Avoid wasting precious time on tasks that can be done at a later stage, such as turning race numbers around. Keep to your plan and stay in control.

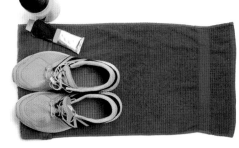

### CHECKLIST

- Towel
- Running shoes
- Nutrition for run
- Water bottle
- Running cap (if hot)

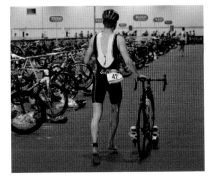

**4 LOCATE YOUR AREA** Find your spot and rack your bike before unclipping your helmet. Always remember that removing your helmet before the bike is racked will lead to disqualification.

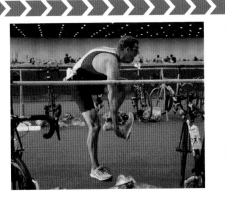

**5 RUNNING SHOES ON** Put on your running shoes (elasticated laces speed up the process). Place your helmet with your other kit, grab your hat, gels, and glasses, and run towards the T2 exit.

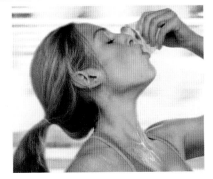

**6 GET RUNNING** There will be plenty of opportunities to get water on the course, so get going as soon as you can. Remember to turn your race number to the front for the run.

**❝** STRAIGHT OFF THE BIKE, YOUR LEGS WILL **FEEL LIKE JELLY**. IT WILL TAKE YOU BETWEEN **100M AND 1KM** TO FIND YOUR **RUNNING LEGS** AND SETTLE INTO A RHYTHM. **❞**

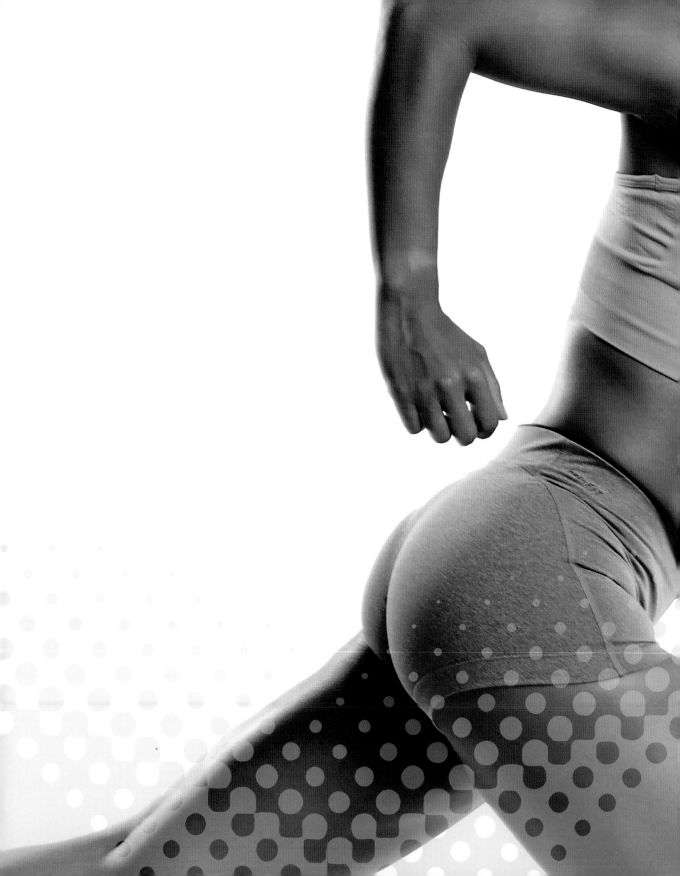

# THE
# RUNNING LAB

# THE RUNNING CYCLE

**Running involves two** main phases. The floating phase, when both feet leave the ground, is divided into toe-off and swing. In the stance phase, divided into strike and support, the body absorbs forces from the ground and stores energy to keep moving itself forwards. Knowing how the body works throughout this cycle will help you perfect your technique, and run faster.

## KEY »

Different muscles work at different stages of the running cycle. Muscles in the lower leg and foot absorb impact and provide power to push off; muscles in the upper leg work to move you forwards; muscles in the trunk keep you stable and balanced, helping you maintain form.

- PECTORALIS MAJOR
- HIP FLEXORS
- GLUTEALS
- ADDUCTORS
- ABDUCTORS
- QUADRICEPS
- HAMSTRINGS
- SOLEUS
- GASTROCNEMIUS

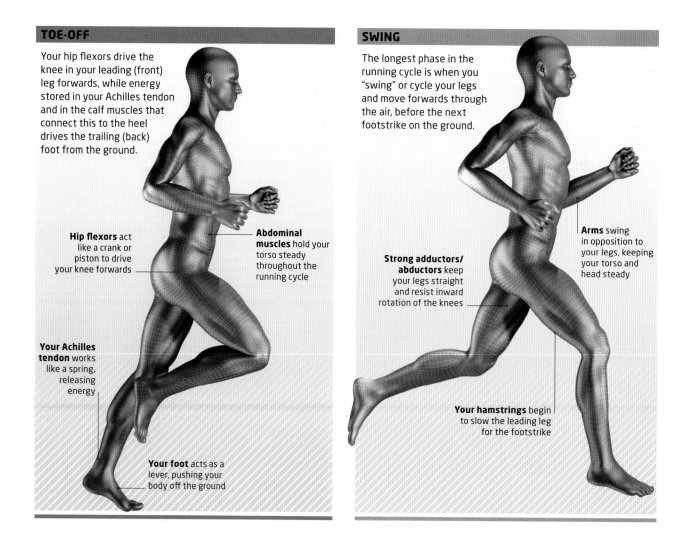

**TOE-OFF**

Your hip flexors drive the knee in your leading (front) leg forwards, while energy stored in your Achilles tendon and in the calf muscles that connect this to the heel drives the trailing (back) foot from the ground.

**Hip flexors** act like a crank or piston to drive your knee forwards

**Abdominal muscles** hold your torso steady throughout the running cycle

**Your Achilles tendon** works like a spring, releasing energy

**Your foot** acts as a lever, pushing your body off the ground

**SWING**

The longest phase in the running cycle is when you "swing" or cycle your legs and move forwards through the air, before the next footstrike on the ground.

**Strong adductors/abductors** keep your legs straight and resist inward rotation of the knees

**Arms** swing in opposition to your legs, keeping your torso and head steady

**Your hamstrings** begin to slow the leading leg for the footstrike

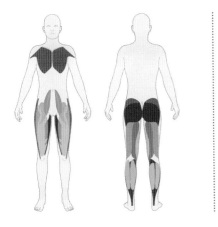

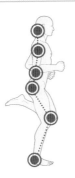

# THE KINETIC CHAIN: RUNNING

Running is the only triathlon discipline in which your body bears all of its own weight, so your kinetic chain (see p.13) needs to be especially robust to reduce the impact and loading force that your joints and bones endure during training and racing. When you get off your bike and head into the final stage of the triathlon, your legs will feel like jelly at first – but a strong kinetic chain will help you power through the run to the finishing line. Strengthening the kinetic chain through better technique and practice will minimize the risk of injury and lessen the load on your body.

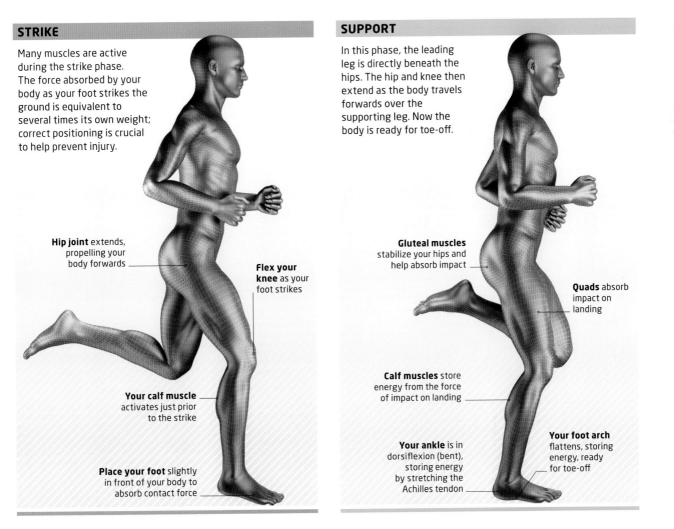

## STRIKE

Many muscles are active during the strike phase. The force absorbed by your body as your foot strikes the ground is equivalent to several times its own weight; correct positioning is crucial to help prevent injury.

**Hip joint** extends, propelling your body forwards

**Flex your knee** as your foot strikes

**Your calf muscle** activates just prior to the strike

**Place your foot** slightly in front of your body to absorb contact force

## SUPPORT

In this phase, the leading leg is directly beneath the hips. The hip and knee then extend as the body travels forwards over the supporting leg. Now the body is ready for toe-off.

**Gluteal muscles** stabilize your hips and help absorb impact

**Quads** absorb impact on landing

**Calf muscles** store energy from the force of impact on landing

**Your ankle** is in dorsiflexion (bent), storing energy by stretching the Achilles tendon

**Your foot arch** flattens, storing energy, ready for toe-off

# FOOTSTRIKE

**To become a better runner**, start at the bottom by looking at how your foot hits the ground. Footstrike styles vary between runners, but there are three broad types and each is found in all levels of runner. Whatever your style, assessing how your foot makes contact with the ground can help you to improve your technique and increase your running efficiency.

## RACING FLATS

Modern supportive training shoes encourage many people who take up running to be heel-strikers. However, many elite distance runners prefer flat, light racing shoes; these promote a forefoot or mid-foot strike that can ultimately lead to a faster run.

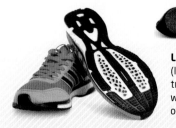

**Lightweight** trainers (left) mimic older-style track shoes (above), which had no support or heel cushioning.

## TESTING STRIKE STYLES

You can start to understand the effects of different strike styles by trying the following simple test:

1 Standing on a hard surface, take off your shoes, rock back on your heels, and take a very small jump. Do your feet hurt? This is similar to the effect of heel strike.

2 Now try rocking forward, with your weight on the front part of the foot, and jump again. The bounce and elasticity that you feel is what forefoot strike runners use to run more efficiently.

Whatever your footstrike, avoid over-striding and landing heavily. If you want to change your strike, do it gradually and under the supervision of a qualified running coach.

## HEEL STRIKE

A heel strike is where the runner's foot lands heel-first on the ground. The foot then rolls forward, placing load through the arch, before finishing with a pushing-off or toeing-off action. Heel striking has become one of the most common forms of footstrike over the past 30–40 years, due to the use of modern training shoes.

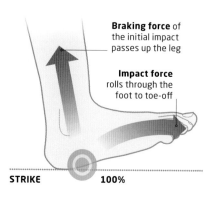

**Braking force** of the initial impact passes up the leg

**Impact force** rolls through the foot to toe-off

STRIKE          100%

## MIDFOOT RUNNING

In mid-foot running, the middle of the runner's foot strikes the ground first, so that the foot is almost parallel to the ground and the arch is loaded on impact. This flat-footed strike means that more force is required to drive the body forwards, and so mid-foot running is not a particularly economical strike.

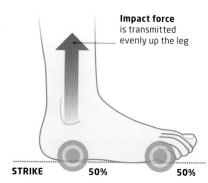

**Impact force** is transmitted evenly up the leg

STRIKE          50%          50%

## FOREFOOT RUNNING

In forefoot running, the ball of the runner's foot strikes the ground first, on its outside edge. The foot then touches down briefly with the heel, rolls slightly inwards, loads, and then toes off. The forefoot strike style can improve running performance and reduce the risk of injury, but it is important not to land with the heel too high as this can place stress on the metatarsal bones.

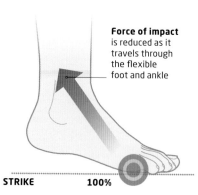

**Force of impact** is reduced as it travels through the flexible foot and ankle

STRIKE          100%

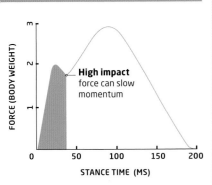

**The heel strike** can create a force of up to two times the body weight. This impact force can lead to injury over time.

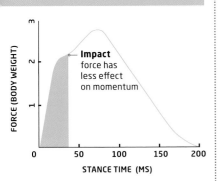

**Midfoot strikes** have large impact forces, but the stress is reduced because the force is spread across the foot.

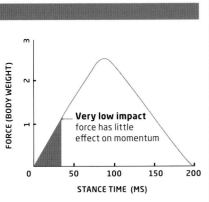

**Forefoot strikes** should result in less force on impact; it is dissipated by the flexibility in the front part of the foot.

## BAREFOOT RUNNING SHOES

Minimalist, or "barefoot", running shoes have thin soles that provide protection from sharp stones without the artificial support or cushioning of standard trainers. The aim is to help promote a "natural" style of running that feels similar to running barefoot. If you run in this way your body can make better use of stored energy, but you will need to have good running technique in order to avoid injury. If you wish to try "barefoot" running, make the change over a period of time, starting with a 30-second run, and progress from there within the 10 per cent rule.

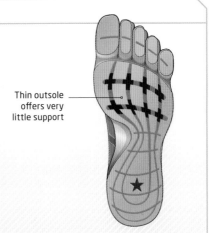

Thin outsole offers very little support

# WHAT YOUR SHOES TELL YOU

The foot and ankle rotate naturally as you run, but the degree of rotation varies between runners. A small amount of rolling inwards (pronation) or outwards (supination) is okay, but if it is more uneven (known as overpronation or underpronation), it can affect your running efficiency and may cause injury. The pattern of wear on your shoes shows how your foot strikes the ground and rotates, and this can help you choose shoes best suited to your running style.

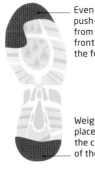

Even push-off from the front of the foot

Weight placed on the centre of the heel

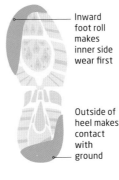

Inward foot roll makes inner side wear first

Outside of heel makes contact with ground

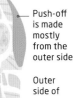

Push-off is made mostly from the outer side

Outer side of heel takes greatest impact

**NORMAL PRONATOR**
A normal pronator's foot rotates 15 per cent when running. The outer heel makes initial contact with the ground, then the whole foot. Stability shoes are good for normal pronators.

**OVERPRONATOR**
If your foot rotates inwards by more than 15 per cent you overpronate. The foot arch tends to be lower. Overpronators may find motion control shoes the best choice.

**UNDERPRONATOR**
If your shoe is worn mainly on the outer side, you underpronate: your foot rotates less than 15 per cent. A shoe with neutral cushioning encourages natural foot motion.

# EFFICIENT RUNNING

**Running well** is about running economically, using less oxygen per step. One of the best ways to develop running speed and endurance is to correct your alignment, specifically around your centre of gravity, in the hip area.

> **"** A **STRONG TRUNK** IS ESSENTIAL TO **MAINTAIN BALANCE.** IT ALSO HELPS MAKE YOUR **BREATHING** MORE **EFFECTIVE** WHEN YOU RUN. **"**

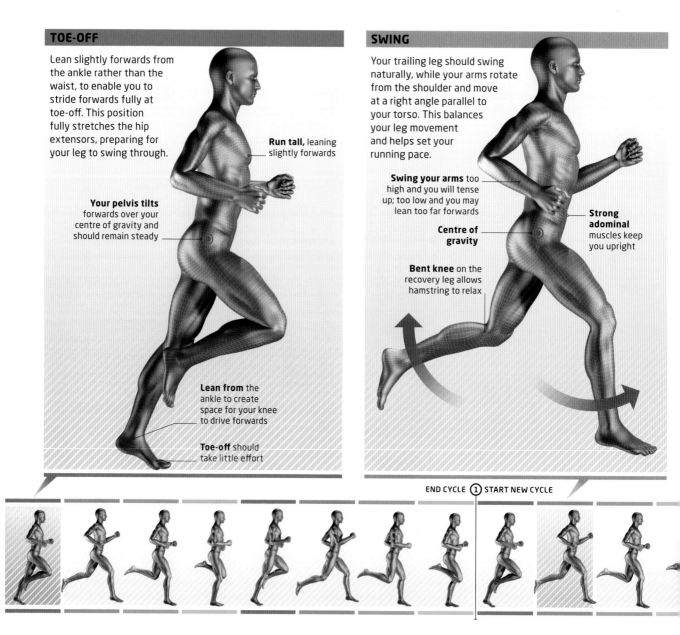

## TOE-OFF

Lean slightly forwards from the ankle rather than the waist, to enable you to stride forwards fully at toe-off. This position fully stretches the hip extensors, preparing for your leg to swing through.

**Run tall,** leaning slightly forwards

**Your pelvis tilts** forwards over your centre of gravity and should remain steady

**Lean from** the ankle to create space for your knee to drive forwards

**Toe-off** should take little effort

## SWING

Your trailing leg should swing naturally, while your arms rotate from the shoulder and move at a right angle parallel to your torso. This balances your leg movement and helps set your running pace.

**Swing your arms** too high and you will tense up; too low and you may lean too far forwards

**Centre of gravity**

**Bent knee** on the recovery leg allows hamstring to relax

**Strong adominal** muscles keep you upright

END CYCLE ① START NEW CYCLE

## KEEP CENTRED

You should keep your body as upright as possible when running, with your hips just behind the point where your foot strikes. Your torso may twist slightly when your legs are driving forwards, but you can minimize this movement by keeping your arms parallel to your body as much as possible. Your arms can move towards your midline, but do not let them cross it, or they will also pull your legs out of alignment. Keep your head relaxed, and look straight ahead, not down.

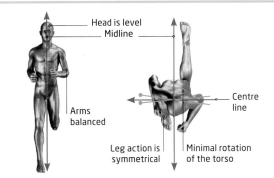

Head is level
Midline
Arms balanced
Centre line
Leg action is symmetrical
Minimal rotation of the torso

## STRIKE

Strike your foot just in front of your centre of gravity. This maintains your forward momentum and allows your leg to absorb the impact force, which is briefly stored as energy, ready to be released later in the cycle.

**Quads** are not at full stretch during the strike phase if the foot is correctly placed under the knee

**Centre of gravity** is just behind the foot

**Your Achilles tendon** stretches, creating about 35 % of the energy for running

**Lower leg** should be as straight as possible

**Strike** parallel to the ground to minimize braking force

## SUPPORT

As you move into midstance and prepare to toe off, keep the upright position but use your knee to lean forwards. This motion moves your body forwards as economically as possible.

**Hold your hands** loosely to prevent tension flowing up your arm

**Centre of gravity** is slightly forward, over your knee

**Calf muscle** should be flexible to allow your Achilles tendon to stretch properly

**Achilles tendon** is ready to release its energy in toe-off

END CYCLE ② START NEW CYCLE

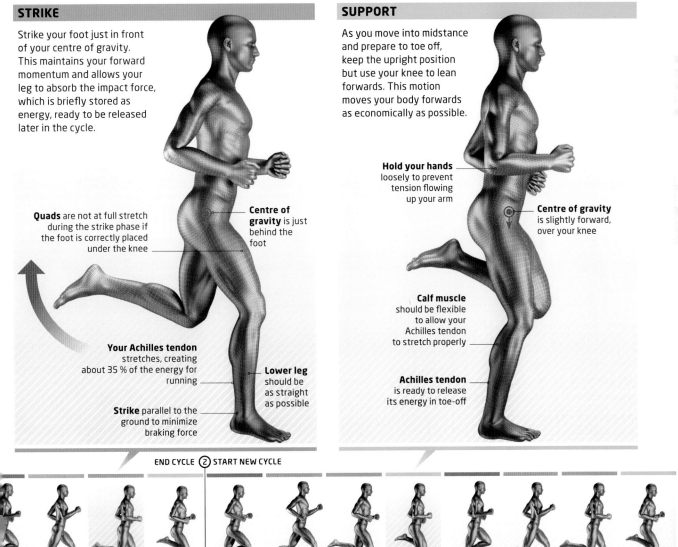

# STRIKE RATE

**An effective way** to run faster is to increase your strike rate, or cadence. This is the number of times one foot hits the ground per minute. Increasing your strike rate is possible no matter which type of footstrike you use, provided you avoid over-striding and landing heavily. Good runners don't hit the ground heavily and linger there; ground contact is quick, light, and virtually silent.

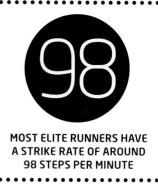

**98**

MOST ELITE RUNNERS HAVE A STRIKE RATE OF AROUND 98 STEPS PER MINUTE

## INCREASING CADENCE

The diagram below shows how your ground contact time fits into the running cycle. it only takes a small increase in your strike rate to run much faster. For example, research suggests that an increase from 170 to 175 steps per minute (counting both feet) can gain about 8m (9yd) per minute. When working on increasing your cadence, aim for an improvement of around 5 per cent at a time.

**KEY »**

● TOE-OFF
● SWING
● STRIKE
● SUPPORT

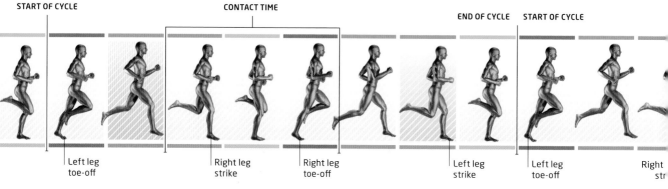

START OF CYCLE          CONTACT TIME                    END OF CYCLE    START OF CYCLE

Left leg toe-off | Right leg strike | Right leg toe-off | Left leg strike | Left leg toe-off | Right str

## WHAT'S MY PACE?

**Whether you have** a specific goal – beating your personal best, for example – or are running your first race, it is essential to know the pace that you are able to run at right now. You just need two pieces of information to calculate your pace: the distance of the run and the time it takes you to complete it. Increasing your strike rate is one of the ways in which you can increase your pace and reach your goal.

**1** **GO TO A RUNNING TRACK** or use a GPS running watch to measure out the distance you are going to run.

**2** **RUN THE DISTANCE** and time yourself accurately with a stopwatch or the GPS running watch.

**3** **CALCULATE YOUR RUNNING PACE** by dividing your time by the distance of the route. Pace is usually expressed as minutes per kilometre or mile.

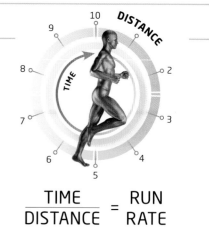

$$\frac{\text{TIME}}{\text{DISTANCE}} = \frac{\text{RUN}}{\text{RATE}}$$

# FORM AND CADENCE

Good form is essential to maintaining and increasing your strike rate; a strong kinetic chain (see p.61) will enable you to increase your cadence and run faster. This diagram shows how form can affect strike rate.

**Incorrect form**
The runner appears to bounce. This is inefficient and will lower the strike rate.

**Arms and torso** twist to the left and right

**Overstriding** will place strike ahead of the centre of gravity

**Knee** is bent to enable leg to recover quickly, ready for the next strike

**Footstrike** is light and quick

**Correct form**
An upright, level running motion will allow an increased strike rate.

**Arms swing** from the shoulders, with minimal sideways movement

**Hips** are stable, not moving from side to side

**Knee** is directly over the foot for stability at high speed

**Braking force** travels up the outstretched leg

## WHAT TO AVOID

### POUNDING
A good pair of running shoes provides great comfort, but some runners develop a heavy footstrike because of the cushioning, and hit the ground with too much force.

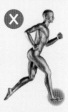

### OVERSTRIDING
A long stride is not always the best. If your feet are striking too far in front of your centre of gravity, this creates a braking force which reduces your running efficiency.

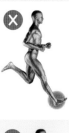

### UNUSED ARMS
Proper arm movement is an important part of good running form. Do not be tempted to minimize arm movement in an effort to focus your energy on the legs.

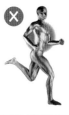

### TWISTING
Twisting occurs when arm movement is both excessive and poorly directed. If the arms swing from side to side, it causes too much lateral movement of the trunk.

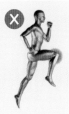

### BOUNCING
It might seem normal to run with a natural bounce to your gait, but this is a waste of valuable energy and momentum. You should aim for a smooth, level motion instead.

### SLOW PACE
Some runners may adopt an overly slow pace in the search for efficiency or to save their energy - in fact, this has the opposite effect, using more energy for lesser results.

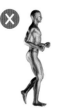

# WARMING UP AND COOLING DOWN

**Training is hard** on the body, and if you're too hasty in the jump from rest to intense exercise and back again, you run the risk of acute injuries and chronic conditions. A good warm-up and cool-down are an essential part of the triathlete's regime.

**66** GOING THROUGH YOUR **REGULAR WARM-UP** PRE-RACE, GETS YOU TUNED IN TO **SOMETHING FAMILIAR** AMIDST ALL THE **NOISE** OF THE COMPETITION ON RACE DAY. **99**

## YOUR ROUTE TO SUCCESS

### PREPARING YOUR BODY

Warming up properly prepares you both physically and mentally for exercise, enabling you to perform at your best from the outset. An inadequate warm-up can lead to poor or inefficient technique, which may result in injuries, not just to your muscles, but also to your joints and ligaments.

There are two main types of warm-up: general and specific. A general warm-up might consist of gentle leg or arm swings to mobilize your shoulder and hip joints, combined with a little light jogging or cycling. A sport-specific warm-up (such as the one for running, opposite) is suitable for more intense training or racing.

Cooling down, or "flushing", is also essential, as it helps you to recover fully and quickly following exercise, and keeps you in optimum shape. Not cooling down properly can lead to stiff and sore muscles.

### PHYSIOLOGICAL BENEFITS

During exercise, your muscles need more energy and oxygen. Warming up increases your breathing, heart rate, and body temperature. This allows your heart to pump a greater amount of oxygenated, nutrient-rich blood into your muscles, while also getting rid of waste by-products such as carbon dioxide. To enable this to happen, the blood vessels in your muscles expand (a process known as "vasodilation"), raising the temperature of your muscles and the speed at which they can relax and contract, which improves the overall efficiency of your movements.

Cooling down after exercise helps to flush away adrenaline and waste by-products such as lactic acid from your muscles, reduces the potential for delayed onset muscle soreness or "DOMS" (see p.155), and returns your heart to its resting rate.

### PSYCHOLOGICAL BENEFITS

Warming up also offers a range of psychological benefits. Knowing that you have prepared your body fully will give you the confidence to train or race hard without fear of injury, while the warm-up itself will help you to clear your mind of distractions and concentrate on the race. Use the warm-up to focus on similar visualization techniques to the ones you have practised in your swim sessions (see pp.20–21). This will make your movements feel more "natural" during each leg of the race.

## HOW DO I WARM UP?

For your running sessions, the warm-up described on pp.70–73 is comprehensive but doesn't require much space to perform: a 100m (330ft) stretch of road or grass is sufficient. If you are warming up prior to a swim or cycle session, then you will need to perform a sport-specific warm-up (see pp.20–21 and p.48).

## HOW SHOULD I STRETCH?

There are two main types of stretch: dynamic and static. Dynamic stretches are movement-based and prepare your muscles for exercise; static stretches are performed when your body is at rest. You should therefore use dynamic stretches in your warm-up and reserve static stretches for cooling down.

## WHAT IS "FLUSHING"?

Intense exercise causes micro-tears in your muscle fibres. Cooling down using static "flushing" stretches (see pp.74–75) helps to repair your muscles by carrying nutrient-rich blood into them and pumping away any toxins. Gently contracting and relaxing your muscles when flushing helps your blood vessels to do this efficiently.

### PREVENTING INJURY

The best way to avoid injury is to prevent it happening in the first place. This is referred to as pre-habilitation (or pre-hab). It includes practising good technique and doing strength and conditioning sessions to ensure that you are strong and robust enough for triathlon and the level at which you want to compete. A good warm-up, too, is a vital part of pre-hab. So too is cooling down (flushing), as it reduces your likelihood of suffering stiffness and soreness, and helps your muscles to get rid of waste products produced during exercise. Pre-hab exercises using a foam roller (see pp.150–153) and regular sports massages can also help to flush blood through the muscles, and keep problem areas from flaring up.

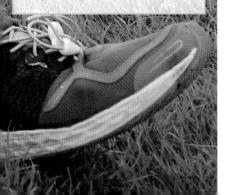

## SAMPLE WARM-UP PROGRAMME

>> **AIM OF PROGRAMME:** TO WARM UP YOUR MUSCLES IN PREPARATION FOR RUNNING

>> **DURATION OF WARM-UP:** 10 MINUTES

| | EXERCISE | SETS | REPS | REST |
|---|---|---|---|---|
| 01 | JOGGING GENTLE | 1 x | 4 (REPEAT 4 TIMES) | 10 SECS |
| 02 | JOGGING MODERATE | 1 x | 4 | 20 SECS |
| 03 | DYNAMIC HAMSTRING STRETCH | 1 x | 10 – WALKING | NONE |
| | | 1 x | 10 – JOGGING | NONE |
| | | 1 x | 10 – CONTINUOUS | NONE |
| 04 | WALKING LUNGE | 1 x | 10 | NONE |
| 05 | CHIROPRACTIC STRETCH | 1 x | 10 | NONE |
| 06 | DYNAMIC GLUTE STRETCH | 1 x | 10 | NONE |
| 07 | DYNAMIC HIP FLEXOR STRETCH | 1 x | 10 | NONE |
| 08 | DYNAMIC REC FEM STRETCH | 1 x | 10 | NONE |
| 09 | ALIGNMENT DRILLS (PUSH & PULL) | 1 x | 1 EACH | NONE |

## SAMPLE COOL-DOWN PROGRAMME

>> **AIM OF PROGRAMME:** TO ENCOURAGE BLOOD CIRCULATION TO THE MUSCLES POST-RUN

>> **DURATION OF COOL-DOWN:** 3-4 MINUTES

| | EXERCISE | SETS | REPS | REST |
|---|---|---|---|---|
| 01 | SOFT BACKWARDS LUNGE | 1 x | 4-6 | NONE |
| 02 | CALF AND HIP FLEXOR FLUSHING | 1 x | 4-6 | NONE |
| 03 | GLUTES FLUSHING | 1 x | 4-6 | NONE |
| 04 | HAMSTRING FLUSHING | 1 x | 4-6 | NONE |

# 01 JOGGING
## GENTLE

Gentle jogging is a great way to start your warm-up: it releases friction-reducing synovial fluid into the joints, increases your heart rate, and stretches out your tendons.

Start with your feet hip-width apart. Gently lean forwards until you feel off-balance, then begin to jog at a gentle pace for 25 steps. Repeat four times, pausing for a few seconds before each repetition.

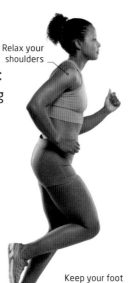

Relax your shoulders

Keep your foot strike light and bouncy

# 02 JOGGING
## MODERATE

Warming up at a moderate speed will give you a feel for timing your stride at race pace, as well as increasing your heart rate and breathing.

Start with your feet hip-width apart. Gently lean forwards, then jog at a moderate pace for 25 steps. Repeat four times, pausing for a few seconds before each repetition.

Drive with your arms

Push forwards with your legs

# 03 DYNAMIC HAMSTRING
## STRETCH

Your hamstrings are the key muscles used in running, so you need to make sure they are properly prepared. Alternate stretching with walking for 10 reps. Speed up to stretching and jogging for a further 10 reps, hopping on one leg as you kick with the other. Finally, alternate sides continuously, with no steps Pin between, for 10 reps.

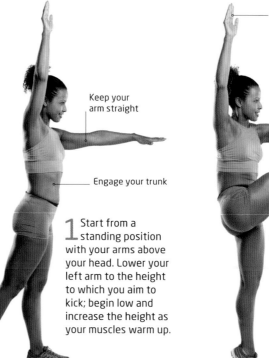

Keep your arm straight

Engage your trunk

1 Start from a standing position with your arms above your head. Lower your left arm to the height to which you aim to kick; begin low and increase the height as your muscles warm up.

Keep your right arm raised for balance

Keep your leg straight with a soft knee

2 Kick your right leg up until your foot touches your left hand. Return your foot to the floor and stretch both arms above your head. Take a few steps forward and repeat the exercise on the other side.

## 04 WALKING LUNGE

This simple, highly effective exercise improves your balance while stretching out the major muscles in your glutes and quadriceps. To make balancing more challenging, place your hands on your head.

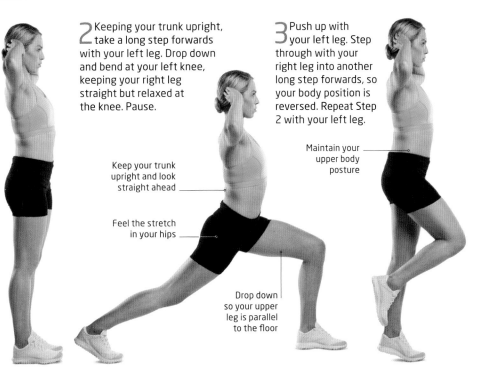

2 Keeping your trunk upright, take a long step forwards with your left leg. Drop down and bend at your left knee, keeping your right leg straight but relaxed at the knee. Pause.

3 Push up with your left leg. Step through with your right leg into another long step forwards, so your body position is reversed. Repeat Step 2 with your left leg.

Maintain your upper body posture

Keep your trunk upright and look straight ahead

Feel the stretch in your hips

Drop down so your upper leg is parallel to the floor

1 Stand with your feet hip-width apart and your hands touching the sides of your head. Ensure that your shoulders, hips, and feet are in line.

## 05 CHIROPRACTIC STRETCH

This exercise flexes and mobilizes your spine; this is particularly important if you spend your working days sitting at a desk. You may hear or feel small pops as your vertebrae realign. Drop your chin onto your chest to get a stronger stretch down your spine.

Maintain a long back and upright torso

Twist your hips in the opposite direction to your upper body

Pull your leg back to kick

1 Start from a standing position and walk forwards at a moderate pace, holding your upper body upright. After a few steps, step forwards with your left leg and swing your arms to your left.

2 Swing your arms and upper body to the right, while kicking your right leg across your body to the left. Straighten out as you lower your leg. Take a few steps and repeat the exercise on the other side.

## 06 DYNAMIC GLUTE STRETCH

Moving a limb through its full range of motion stretches your muscles dynamically, increasing core muscle temperature in preparation for exercise. This stretch will also loosen off any tightness you may have in and around your glutes.

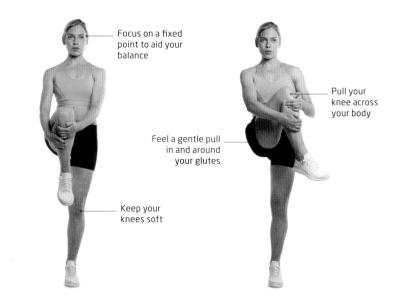

Focus on a fixed point to aid your balance

Pull your knee across your body

Feel a gentle pull in and around your glutes

Keep your knees soft

1 Start from a standing position. Lift your right leg up to hip height, bending your knee. Hold the front of your right leg with both hands.

2 Using both hands, gently draw your right knee across your body and slightly up towards your left shoulder. Lower your leg to the ground, take a few steps forwards, and repeat on the opposite side.

## 07 DYNAMIC HIP FLEXOR STRETCH

This exercise loosens and opens your chest muscles and hip flexors. Your hip flexors are used in all three triathlon disciplines, and can be the source of lower-back pain or injury if they're not stretched properly.

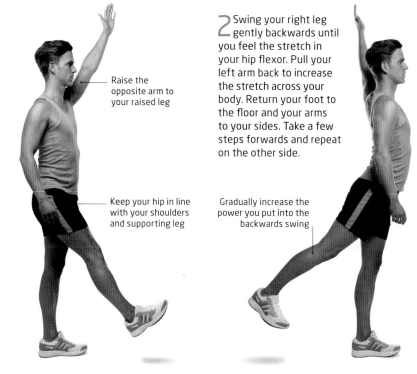

Raise the opposite arm to your raised leg

Keep your hip in line with your shoulders and supporting leg

2 Swing your right leg gently backwards until you feel the stretch in your hip flexor. Pull your left arm back to increase the stretch across your body. Return your foot to the floor and your arms to your sides. Take a few steps forwards and repeat on the other side.

Gradually increase the power you put into the backwards swing

1 Start from a standing position with your right leg off the ground, your left leg slightly bent, and your left arm raised above your head. Kick your right leg gently forwards in a pendulum-like swing.

# 08 DYNAMIC REC FEM STRETCH

The "rec fem" (rectus femoris) is part of the quads at the front of your thighs, and plays a key role during the swing phase of the running cycle (see pp.60-61). It has a tendency to become quite tight; keeping your rec fem flexible will help you open your hips while running and prevent injury.

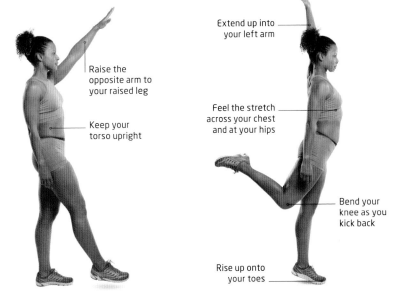

Raise the opposite arm to your raised leg

Keep your torso upright

Extend up into your left arm

Feel the stretch across your chest and at your hips

Bend your knee as you kick back

Rise up onto your toes

**1** Start from a standing position with your right foot off the ground, your left leg bent slightly at the knee, and your left arm raised above your head. Kick your right leg gently forwards.

**2** Swing your leg to kick back towards your buttocks, while also stretching your left arm up and back. Repeat on the other side.

# 09 ALIGNMENT DRILLS

You will need a partner for these two drills. They will help you understand how your body should feel when it's correctly aligned for running.

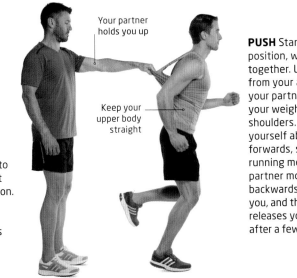

Your partner holds you up

Keep your upper body straight

Your partner pushes back to hold your weight

Drive your arms forwards and backwards

**PULL** Start in a standing position, with your feet together. Lean forwards from your ankles, letting your partner hold you up by gripping your running top. As you feel yourself begin to topple forwards, set off in a running motion. Your partner moves with you for a few steps, then releases you into a run.

**PUSH** Start in a standing position, with your feet together. Lean forwards from your ankles, letting your partner support your weight at the shoulders. As you feel yourself about to topple forwards, set off in a running motion. Your partner moves backwards with you, and then releases you after a few steps.

# COOLING DOWN

Gently contracting and relaxing muscles – known as "flushing" – will help circulate blood into your fatigued muscles. Keep moving in between these exercises to prevent your muscles from seizing up.

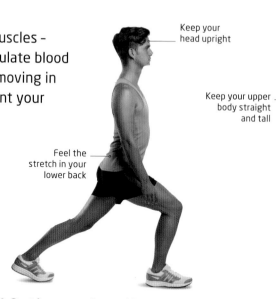

Keep your head upright

Keep your upper body straight and tall

Feel the stretch in your lower back

## 01 SOFT BACKWARDS LUNGE

Start your cool-down by using this lunge to flush your quads, glutes, and hip flexors. The lunge also provides a gentle stretch around your lower back and Achilles tendon.

1 Start from a standing position. Gently step backwards with your left leg, just far enough to exert pressure through your left glute and quad. Keep your weight on your right leg. Engage your abdominals.

2 Pause, then straighten your back and step back into the start position. Take a few steps forwards, shaking out your legs a little as you do so. Repeat on the other side.

## 02 CALF AND HIP FLEXOR FLUSHING

Your calves and hip flexors take much of the load when you run; this flushing exercise will ease off these muscles by gently elongating the muscle fibres.

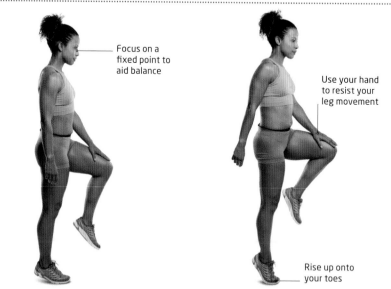

Focus on a fixed point to aid balance

Use your hand to resist your leg movement

Rise up onto your toes

1 Start from a standing position, with your hands loosely at your sides and your upper body tall. Bring your left knee up towards hip height and place your left hand on your raised thigh.

2 Press down with your left hand while pushing up through your raised thigh to counterbalance it. Lean forwards, take a few steps, and repeat on the other side.

## 03 **GLUTES**
## FLUSHING

The glutes help propel you forwards during a run, as well as supporting body alignment. Applying pressure to your glutes while also resisting the movement elongates the muscle fibres and encourages blood circulation.

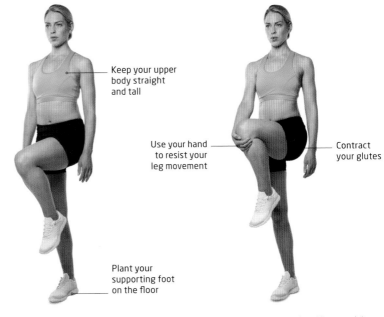

Keep your upper body straight and tall

Use your hand to resist your leg movement

Contract your glutes

Plant your supporting foot on the floor

1 Start from a standing position, with your hands loosely at your sides and your upper body tall. Raise your left knee towards hip height.

2 Take hold of your raised knee with your right hand. Push out to the left with your hand while pushing back with your knee. Return to the start position and repeat on the opposite side.

## 04 **HAMSTRING**
## FLUSHING

For the first few times you flush your hamstrings - especially after running - make sure you stretch them very gently, as they can have a tendency to cramp.

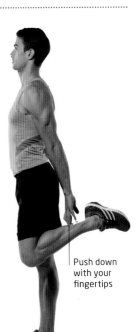

2 Reach down with the fingers of your left hand and press gently down on your heel. Push your heel upwards to counterbalance the pressure. You can also move your knee a little forwards or backwards to loosen off different parts of the hamstrings. Return to the start position and repeat on the opposite side.

Keep your body in a straight line from shoulder to knee

Push down with your fingertips

1 Start from a standing position, with your hands loosely at your sides and your upper body tall. Bend your left knee and kick your heel up towards your buttocks.

# RUN SESSIONS

**Running in a triathlon** is very different from competing in a typical running race. After the bike, you start this final leg already fatigued; if you are new to triathlon, and you've overdone it on the bike, you may find you need to walk for a while. Running is a weight-bearing discipline, so you must hold good form to get through the run and across the finish line. Training at the different levels below allows you to hone your technique and gradually progress to achieving more challenging goals without putting undue strain on your body.

❝ HOLDING **GOOD FORM** AND JUDGING **YOUR PACE** DURING THE FINAL STAGE OF THE RACE IS CRUCIAL IF YOU WANT TO GET THE MOST OUT OF YOUR **TRIATHLON PERFORMANCE**. BEAR THIS IN MIND THROUGHOUT YOUR RUNNING SESSIONS. ❞

## TRAINING LEVELS 1–5

### 1 EASY

Long steady distance (LSD) pace can be about building endurance, or it can be used for recovery over a shorter distance. These runs are best done on grass to lower the chance of injury. It's easy to lose concentration at this pace; building good form is key.

**TARGET:** 50–60 per cent of maximum heart rate (HR max).

**MAIN SET:** Aim for a steady run for 30 minutes (for sprint distance), up to 3 hours (Ironman).

**RECOVERY:** Ease off to a gentle jog before completing cool-down stretches (see pp.74–75).

**PROGRESSION:** Increase distance by 10 per cent with every run until you reach race distance.

**BENEFITS:** LSD running is about increasing your aerobic efficiency (enabling your body to use oxygen at increasingly higher speeds) and teaching the body to use fat as fuel (see pp.90–91 and p.160).

### 2 TEMPO

Tempo running is about increasing the speed, and it feels more rhythmic. It is a little faster than LSD running, so you will become fatiguing over time.

**TARGET:** 60–70 per cent of HR max.

**MAIN SET:** Complete in sequence:
• Start with an easy 5-minute jog, then accelerate your pace to a speed that feels like 75 per cent effort
• Hold the speed and effort for 15–20 minutes
Gradually reduce your speed for a 5-minute easy run warm-down.

**RECOVERY:** Along with the easing down into a jog, finish with some flushing (see pp.69, 74–75).

**PROGRESSION:** Aim to increase the length of time you run at a higher speed (e.g. up to 1 hour), but always ensure it is controlled and sustained.

**BENEFITS:** Tempo running gives you more of a feeling of speed, while still building aerobic capacity (see p.160).

### 3 THRESHOLD

This is race pace work, and will teach you to run with increased economy and hold form as you fatigue.

**TARGET:** 70–85 per cent of HR max; will feel stressful after 5–10 minutes.

**MAIN SET:** Choose one of these sets:
• 1–3 x 15-minute runs, jog for 1 minute or until HR down to 130 beats per minute (bpm), OR
• 2–4 x 1 mile, recovery jog between sets for 1 minute, jog for 1 minute or until HR down to 130bpm, OR
• 1–3 x 10–12 minute runs, jog for 1 minute or until HR down to 130bpm

**RECOVERY:** Flushing (see pp.74–75).

**PROGRESSION:** As you learn to handle the discomfort that comes with a harder level of training, your ability to run faster for longer will improve.

**BENEFITS:** Increases your feel for race-pace pressure and rhythm; good for dissipating higher levels of lactate production (see p.160).

## SAMPLE SESSION

This table shows you how to structure a session around your main set at Levels 3-5. The levels below offer a choice of run sets. Focus on key areas to improve and aim to complete three different run sessions per week. Once you know your strengths and weaknesses, you can tailor your training plan to match. *For a sample foundation programme of weekly sessions, see pp.122-123.*

| L3 OR ABOVE | SAMPLE ACTIVITY |
| --- | --- |
| WARM-UP | 10-15 minutes walking/jogging at L3 or above: see warm-up on p.70 |
| PRE-MAIN DRILL SET | 5-10 minutes dynamic stretches: go through warm-up drills on pp.70-73 |
| MAIN SET | Choose a main set from L3: check distance and strike rate throughout |
| COOL-DOWN | Walk until your HR is down, then go through flushing (see pp.74-75) |

## 4 vVO2 MAX

These are intense workouts that can be sustained for short periods of time, about 6-12 minutes.

**TARGET:** 85-96 per cent of HR max; you should not feel the pressure until around 2 minutes into the repetition.

**MAIN SET:** Choose one of these sets:
- 2-3 x 6-12 minutes, OR
- 8-12 x 600m (660yd), 400m (440yd) jog recovery between sets OR
- 2 minutes, 1 minute jog recovery/ 1 minute, 30 seconds jog recovery/ 30 seconds, 30 seconds jog recovery; repeat entire set 4-6 times

**RECOVERY:** Gentle jog of the same duration as the elapsed run time.

**PROGRESSION:** As your fitness and lactate threshold increase (see p.160), aim to complete the maximum number of repetitions (reps) per set.

**BENEFITS:** Improved economy of motion, increased maximal oxygen consumption, and improved lactate tolerance (see p.160).

## 5 MAXIMAL

These run sessions are designed to improve running strength, economy, and speed.

**TARGET:** 96-100 per cent of HR max. Try not to run when tired or lose form during the repetitions.

**MAIN SET:** Choose one of these sets:
- 10-16 x 200m (220yd), OR
- 6-8 x 400m (440yd), recovery 400m (440yd) jog, OR
- 200m (220yd), recovery 200m (220yd)/400m (440yd), recovery 400m (440yd)/600m (660yd), recovery 600m (660yd) - repeat entire set again

**RECOVERY:** Full recovery is needed before another intense session.

**PROGRESSION:** Increase the pace of each sprint; retain recovery time.

**BENEFITS:** Builds strength and adds power. Very useful if you need a sprint finish in your race.

For more details on how Levels 1-5 target physiology and fitness, see pp.160-161.

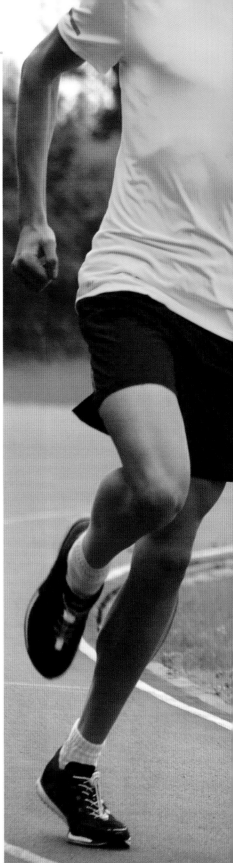

# ASSESSING YOUR RUN FITNESS

**Running can put** a lot of strain on your joints, so a good running technique is essential to limit the impact of this on your body. It is also important to assess your fitness before you begin training, and to review it as your training progresses. This will enable you to work at the right intensity, avoiding the risk of injury through overtraining, or making limited gains due to insufficient training.

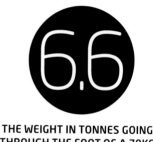

**6.6**

THE WEIGHT IN TONNES GOING THROUGH THE FOOT OF A 70KG (154LB) PERSON RUNNING AT 95 STEPS PER MINUTE

## IS MY GENERAL FITNESS IMPORTANT?

General fitness affects performance in all sports, especially in running, which is an aerobically intensive exercise. Running demands good overall health, so a visit to your doctor for a check-up should be your first move. After that, you can try the basic fitness tests on pp.28–29. If you aren't in particularly good shape, don't push yourself too hard at first. Remember, training is most effective when it is built up steadily, so be content to work up from your current levels.

## HOW DO I CHECK MY AEROBIC FITNESS?

You can find your aerobic fitness by doing a VO2 max test. Your VO2 max is a measure of how much oxygen your body can take in and use while exercising at maximum capacity - in other words, going flat-out. The higher your VO2 max, the fitter you are. Elite distance runners typically have very high VO2 max scores. There are many ways to assess your VO2 max, from simple tests that use gym-based equipment to more scientifically accurate methods. If you are testing your VO2 max for your performance in a specific sport, you should use tests that correlate closely to the sport. For example, the treadmill test and the Cooper 12-minute test, shown opposite, are ideal for runners. Use their corresponding formulas and the tables on pp.158–161 to assess your current fitness and VO2 max score. There are also a number of online converters for the different types of VO2 test. Simply enter your test results into one of these for a quick answer. Retest yourself every 8–12 weeks: you should see your scores climbing.

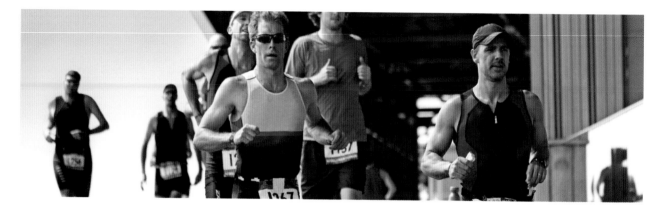

## TAKE THE TREADMILL TEST

This simple test uses a treadmill, which can be found in most gyms. The idea is to run at a fixed pace, slightly increasing the incline of the treadmill every minute until you cannot continue. To carry out the test safely and get accurate results, ask an assistant to increase the incline for you as you run.

### WHAT TO DO

1 **Warm-up** Set the treadmill to a speed of 11.3km/hour (7.02mph) with a flat (0-degree) incline. Use this configuration to warm up for about 10 minutes.

2 **Start the test** When you are ready, ask your assistant to start timing. Using the chart below as a guide, get them to increase the incline every minute.

3 **Stopping** When you can no longer continue, let your assistant know it is time to stop the treadmill and the timer.

### WHAT TO RECORD
• How long you managed to run for

### HOW DO YOU RATE?
Top male athletes tend to have VO2 max rates in the 60s, 70s, and 80s, and top female athletes in the 50s, 60s, and 70s. Depending on age, for people of average fitness, VO2 max tends to range from around 30 to 50 in men, and the high 20s to the mid-40s for women (see p.158).

| TIME (MINUTES) | 0 | 1 | 2 | 3 | 4 | 5 | 6 | 7 | 8 | 9 | 10 | 11 | 12 | 13 | 14 | 15 |
|---|---|---|---|---|---|---|---|---|---|---|---|---|---|---|---|---|
| SLOPE | 0° | 2° | 4° | 6° | 8° | 10° | 11° | 12° | 13° | 14° | 15° | 16° | 17° | 18° | 19° | 20° |

$$\text{VO2 MAX} = 2 + (\text{TIME}^* \times 2)$$

*TIME = the total time of the test in minutes and fractions of a minute

## TRY THE COOPER 12-MINUTE TEST

This test was developed in 1968 by Dr Ken Cooper, inventor of aerobics. It's best done on a 400m (400 yd) track, but you can do it wherever you can record distance. If you don't own a GPS watch, you'll need an assistant.

### WHAT TO DO

1 **Warm-up** After a 10-minute warm-up, tell your assistant you're ready.

2 **Start the test** Your assistant starts the timer and you set off. At the end of each lap, your assistant shouts how much time you have left.

3 **Stopping** After 12 minutes, your assistant halts the test and records the distance.

### WHAT TO RECORD
• How far you ran in 12 minutes

### HOW DO YOU RATE?
In 12 minutes, most men with good fitness levels can run over 2,000m (6,562ft) and women more than 1,700m (5,577ft). (See p.159.)

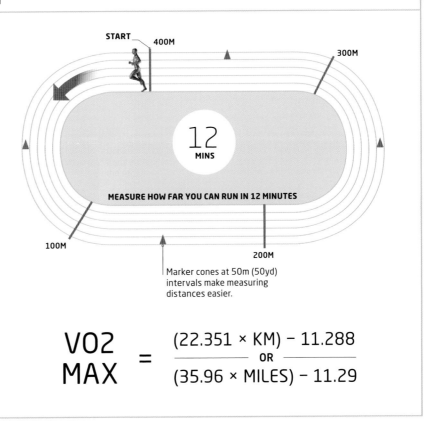

START 400M 300M

**12 MINS**

MEASURE HOW FAR YOU CAN RUN IN 12 MINUTES

100M 200M

Marker cones at 50m (50yd) intervals make measuring distances easier.

$$\text{VO2 MAX} = \frac{(22.351 \times \text{KM}) - 11.288}{(35.96 \times \text{MILES}) - 11.29} \text{ OR}$$

# VARY YOUR RUNNING

**Consistency in training** is crucial, but it is also important to add variety to your routine to avoid getting bored. Including some more challenging training sessions in your programme will not only help to improve your fitness and strength but will also keep you motivated.

**" VARYING THE SURFACE** YOU RUN ON ALLOWS YOU TO CLOSELY MATCH THE TYPE OF **TERRAIN** AND **CONDITIONS** YOU MAY FACE ON **RACE DAY. "**

## YOUR ROUTE TO SUCCESS

### RUNNING OFF

When you start running after riding your bike, your legs will probably feel like jelly, especially during longer-distance races such as Ironman or 70.3 (Half Ironman). Practising running off the bike will help reduce the time it takes your legs to adjust and find their rhythm after a long, hard session; it also gets you used to putting your trainers on quickly, which will speed you up in transition. During your first few run-offs, it may take you at least 10-15 minutes to "find your legs", but it will get easier with practice.

### HILL RUNNING

Hill running is a great way to develop mental toughness and strength endurance (the ability to exercise with resistance over some distance), especially when running up long, moderate inclines that seem to go on for miles. It will also help to strengthen your running muscles - your leg muscles are forced to contract more quickly than normal as they have to overcome gravity to get you up the slope. Hill running over a variety of different gradients is also a good way to improve your lactate tolerance (see pp.160-161). As you run up a sharp, steep incline, lactate accumulates in your bloodstream; as the slope flattens and you are running at (or just below) race pace, the lactate will start to dissipate. Running at lactate-threshold trains your body to use oxygen more efficiently and ultimately enables you to run faster.

### FARTLEK

Fartlek (meaning "speed play" in Swedish) refers to a type of training in which you run at different speeds and levels of intensity to add variety to your workouts and improve your stamina. During a 30-minute Fartlek session, for example, you might run for 1 minute at Level 5 then jog for 5 minutes, then run again for 2 minutes at Level 4 and jog for 4 minutes, and so on (see pp.76-77). You can jog and sprint whenever you feel like it and experiment with different times and levels - the main thing is to keep the session varied and have fun with it.

## FOOTWEAR

Whatever surface you run on, you need to ensure you're wearing the correct shoes:

- Track – track spikes or racing flats
- Cross country – cross country spikes or trail shoes
- Off road – trail shoes
- On road – trainers or racing flats
- Sand – bare feet or light trainers
- Hills – trainers or racing flats

## MAKING PROGRESS

As your training progresses, you can start including more difficult workouts into your training programme. However, it is important that you listen to your body and build up to them gradually. By all means, keep challenging yourself and dig deep – but don't step up your training by more than 10 per cent a week.

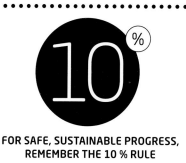

**10 %**

**FOR SAFE, SUSTAINABLE PROGRESS, REMEMBER THE 10 % RULE**

## TEMPO TRAINING

Tempo workouts are run at a pace that you could maintain comfortably for about an hour. They are less difficult than a threshold run but require more effort than a Level 1 run (see p.76). Try to keep a steady rhythm during your workout as your heart rate will start to climb if you push yourself beyond tempo pace.

## YASSO 800s

Yasso 800s (created by US runner Bart Yasso) refers to a type of interval training and fitness testing. The theory is that you can predict your marathon time based on how long it takes you to run 800m (half a mile). For example, if you run 800m in 3 minutes, 18 seconds, your predicted marathon time would be 3 hours, 18 minutes. For the prediction to be more accurate, you would need to run 10 intervals of 800m. Your recovery jog, in between the 800s, should be the same duration as each interval. It is not an exact science and results can vary widely, but some athletes find it a useful way to predict their aerobic capacity and efficiency over the marathon distance.

## BIKE SESSION

A brick session is a form of training where you go from one discipline straight into another. It is used to simulate race-day experience and get your body used to changing sports quickly. Practising transitions ahead of a race will also save you valuable time on the day. Brick sessions might include a swim-to-bike workout or a bike-to-run workout, or even a combination of all three disciplines. You can incorporate different times and levels of intensity into your workouts, but it's a good idea to base your sessions on what you are going to do in your next race.

# WHAT TO WEAR

**As with your swimming** and cycling gear, your running clothes should be comfortable, lightweight, and suitable for all weather conditions. Choosing the right footwear can make a huge difference to your performance, so make sure that your shoes and socks fit properly and do not cause blisters.

**15%**

RACING FLATS HAVE ABOUT 15% LESS CUSHIONING THAN REGULAR TRAINERS

### CAN I TRAIN IN ORDINARY CLOTHES?

If your budget can stretch to it, choose specialist running clothes made from high-tech fabrics that "wick" sweat away from the skin (see p.55). You can train in regular workout gear, but avoid baggy cotton clothes as they absorb sweat and rub the skin, causing soreness and "runner's nipple". Wear double-layered running socks to prevent blisters, though avoid socks made of cotton.

For women, it is essential to have a well-fitting sports bra. Running is a high-impact activity and inadequate support can lead to backache. Get expert help to ensure you have the right size.

### WHAT SHOULD I WEAR IN HOT WEATHER?

In very hot weather, your best option is to run in a T-shirt (or vest) and shorts. If you are not sure how hot it is going to be, start off in a warmer top - you can always take it off if you get too hot. Choose a running top made from breathable fabric that will conduct sweat away from your skin. Make sure you apply a high-factor sunscreen, and wear a peaked cap and sunglasses. Sports socks made from breathable fabric will prevent your feet from getting too clammy.

### WHAT SHOULD I WEAR IN COLD WEATHER?

You will usually need only one layer on your legs as your leg muscles will generate heat as you run. On your upper body, you need layers: wicking fabric next to your skin, then a warmer layer on top. Tops should be long-sleeved and close-fitting. In wet weather, wear a water-resistant, breathable outer jacket to allow moisture to escape.

You lose heat through your head, so wear a thermal hat made of fleece material (or a headband to keep your ears warm). Cover exposed skin with petroleum jelly to protect from the cold and wind, and use sunscreen on bright days; your skin can suffer from the sun's rays even in cool weather. Winter evenings are dark, so wear clothes with visible reflective stripes.

### SHOULD I RUN IN SUPPORTIVE TRAINERS?

Most runners who use the correct footstrike technique (see p.67) will not need supportive trainers - the muscles, tendons, ligaments, and fascia in your feet provide you with a natural support structure. If you have problems with your feet, or you have an unbalanced gait, it is a good idea to consult a medical specialist for advice. A podiatrist may be able to suggest ways to strengthen your feet's natural support system to avoid having to rely on orthotics.

### WHAT ELSE DO I NEED?

Use your training sessions to experiment with energy gels and hydration (see pp.90-93). Working out how much water and nutrition you will need in advance will help you better prepare for race day (see pp.142-145). Carry water in a grip bottle, belt pack, or marathon vest so that you can rehydrate on the go, and take energy gels for longer runs. In poor light, remember to wear clip-on lights to make yourself more visible to traffic.

# THE WELL-EQUIPPED RUNNER

A good running outfit should be lightweight, breathable, and close-fitting. Running clothes can be stylish but you should always go for function over appearance.

**HEADBAND**
Keeps your ears warm and your hair back

**BASE LAYER**
Wear moisture-wicking fabric next to the skin

**GLOVES**
Extremities get cold as body heat is pumped to core muscles

**WATER-RESISTANT JACKET**
Choose breathable fabric with a zip so you can regulate your temperature

**LEGGINGS**
Make sure they are breathable and a close fit

**TRAINERS**
Running is high-impact so always wear appropriate shoes

## CHOOSING YOUR SHOES

### WHERE SHOULD I SHOP?
Always go to a specialist running shop and ask an expert for advice. It is important that your shoes not only fit the shape of your foot, but suit your running style and intensity. Some running shops have treadmills so that a specialist fitter can assess your gait. For the most accurate fit, go shopping after a run, or late in the afternoon, as your feet expand during the day, and wear your normal running socks.

### HOW SHOULD I TEST THEM?
Comfort is key. You should be able to walk normally in your running shoes, without changing your gait. A good sports shop will allow you to run for a few metres in the shoes to try them out. Check that the shoe does not feel tight and that your foot is not moving around in it. Ensure that you are completely happy with the fit before you buy - uncomfortable shoes can be an expensive mistake.

### THE SCIENCE OF "FLATS"
Many experienced runners wear light trainers for regular workouts, and ultra-light "racing flats" for the race itself. Racing flats are built for speed and have minimal support and cushioning. However, they do require correct technique or they may cause injury - novice runners who wish to try them should adapt gradually, using shoes with increasingly less padding.

### CHOOSING THE IDEAL TRAINER
Light trainers are a good compromise between trainers and racing flats. Look for the features described here and make sure the shoes are a good fit before you buy.

**Heel** should be supple so as not to rub on your Achilles tendon

**Cushioning** is low so as not to rub on your ankle

**Toe box** should feel snug - excess movement causes blisters and black toenails

**Light, flexible sole** gives you a good feel for the ground

**Small heel-to-toe drop** promotes a natural stride

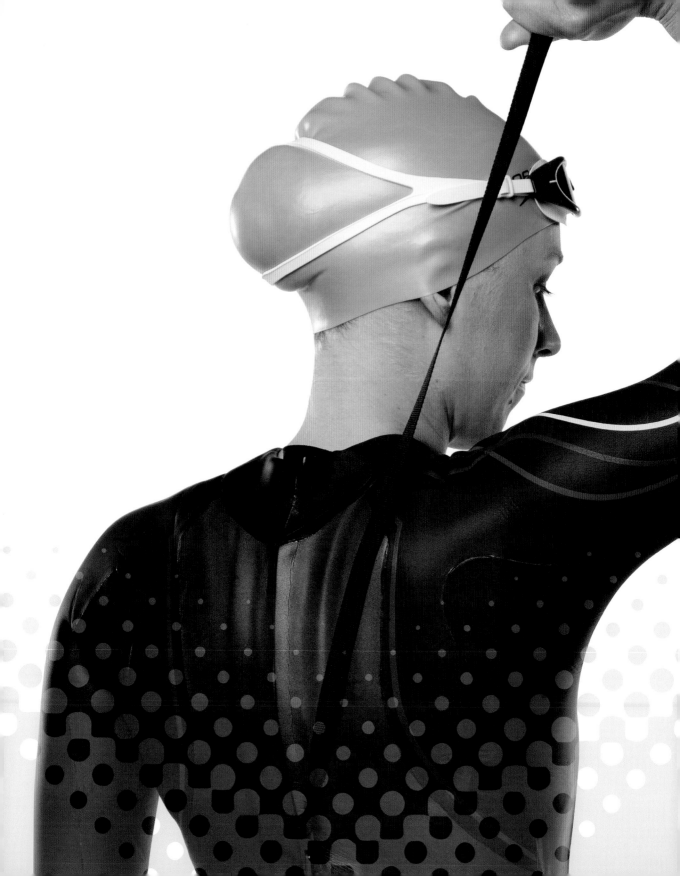

# GETTING STARTED

# YOUR GOALS

**Before you start training,** think about what you want to achieve. Your training will benefit greatly from forward planning and clear objectives. If you include as a discipline learning to transition from from one event to the next, you have four different disciplines to master in triathlon – that's enough to make anyone feel confused about what they should be aiming for. Once you've established your basic fitness levels in swimming, cycling, and running, you can set yourself goals that are challenging and inspiring, but also realistic.

  **❝** ALWAYS **STATE YOUR GOALS AS POSITIVES.** DON'T SAY 'DON'T' AND NEVER SAY 'NEVER'. **SETTING GOALS IS** NOT ABOUT THE BAD THINGS YOU WANT TO AVOID – IT'S **ABOUT THE GOOD THINGS** YOU WANT TO ACHIEVE. **❞**

## YOUR ROUTE TO SUCCESS

### SET GOALS FOR MOTIVATION

Setting goals is a terrific motivator. It's easy to lose focus on vague aims, such as "I want to get fit", so give yourself concrete goals to work towards. Write down specific plans and pin them up somewhere so that you see them every day. You'll get great satisfaction ticking off the goals as you achieve them.

### VARY YOUR GOALS

You can divide your goals into three broad categories: outcome, performance, and process goals.

Outcome goals are those that initially inspire us, but which we don't have total control over and can't guarantee we'll achieve, such as wanting to win a particular race or become an Olympic athlete.

Performance goals are within our full control: they're specific targets, such as reducing times or increasing distances, which you can measure and improve upon.

The most helpful are process goals. They outline what you intend to do to achieve your performance goals; for example, "I will swim at least three times every week".

### SPREAD OUT YOUR GOALS

To keep your motivation and commitment levels high, spread your goals over a period of time, so that you have a range of short-, medium-, and long-term targets.

A short-term goal can be as simple as "I will set my alarm and get to swimming twice this week".

Medium-term goals, especially if they are performance-based, will usually require a phase or two of training, rest, and adaptation. It may take up to two months before you can meet these challenges

Longer-term goals may be years down the road: if you are new to triathlon, it will probably take you about three years to fully master the four disciplines.

# SMART GOALS

Before you set your goals, check them against the SMART criteria shown below. If your goal is SMART, you're on the right track.

| | SPECIFIC | MEASURABLE | ACHIEVABLE | RELEVANT | TIMED |
|---|---|---|---|---|---|
| **CRITERIA** | Define your goals in clear, unambiguous terms. What, specifically, do you want to achieve? And what, precisely, will you have to do to achieve it? | When you set targets, make sure there's an easy way of measuring your progress towards them and of telling when you've achieved your goals. | By all means challenge yourself, but aim for something that's within your reach so you don't end up disappointed and discouraged. | Every goal must serve the purpose of making you the best triathlete you can be. Short- and medium-term goals should all contribute to your long-term goals. | Being vague about when you want to achieve something by isn't helpful. Give yourself realistic deadlines so you can work towards meeting them. |
| **EXAMPLE** | I will go swimming at 5.30am twice per week. | I'll cycle an Ironman course at 68–78 per cent FTP. | I will increase my cadence by 5 steps per minute. | I'll do resistance work to improve my run technique. | I will sort out a swimming coach within three weeks. |
| | I will get coaching to improve my swim stroke. | I will swim at least 7.5km (4.5 miles) per week. | I will shorten my swim time by 10 per cent. | I will swim longer reps to increase my endurance. | I will check my bike fitness within the next month. |

## MAKE THE GOALS YOURS

Be wary of comparing youself to others and trying to compete with them, as this may lead you to set goals that depend on things outside your control. Don't worry about anyone else. It's your triathlon, so set personal goals that will bring out the best in you. People make mistakes; if you didn't get out of bed for that swim or missed a session, it is a waste of time to beat yourself up. Give yourself a positive talking-to, re-set the target, and get back on with it, with a smile.

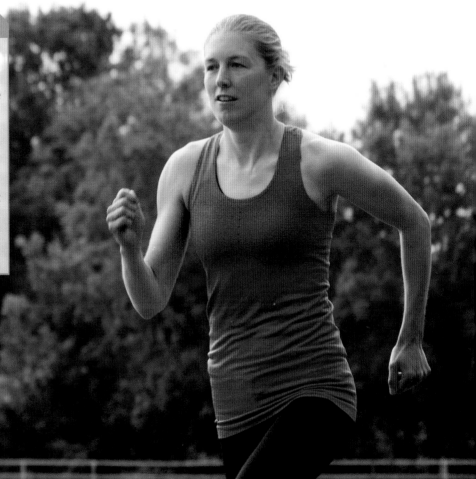

# NUTRITION ESSENTIALS

**Eating the right food** during training is the key to success for triathletes. A well-balanced and nutritious diet will improve your performance, assist your recovery, and help you to avoid injury. Aim to eat healthy and varied meals in sensible quantities. If you fill up on wholesome foods, you will be less likely to hit the calorific snacks after a hard training session. Plan your meals throughout the day and always have healthy snacks on hand to keep your energy levels up.

## HOW TO EAT

- Eat little and often to keep blood sugar balanced throughout the day
- Concentrate on foods with a low glycaemic index (GI: see pp.90-91) and choose healthy, unprocessed snacks, such as fresh fruit
- Have protein-based meals with vegetables or salad in the evening
- Cut back on processed foods and alcoholic drinks
- If using sports drinks, factor in their high sugar content when planning the rest of your day's diet
- Don't eat if you're not hungry

## VITAMINS AND MINERALS

To keep your body working in top condition, it is important to follow a diet rich in vitamins and minerals. A healthy balanced diet (see opposite) will provide most of the vitamins and minerals you need to ensure peak performance and avoid weakness, fatigue, and injury. Supplements can be taken if you are unable to eat certain foods due to allergies or religious requirements, although they should be used as an addition to your diet rather than a replacement. The key is to keep the diet varied; eat a wide range of natural foods to make sure you get all the vitamins and minerals available. If in doubt, consult a sports nutritionist for advice.

| NUTRIENT | PURPOSE | GOOD SOURCES |
|----------|---------|--------------|
| CALCIUM | Promotes healthy bone development, regulates muscle contractions, supports blood clotting. | Dairy products, leafy greens, tofu, fortified flour, soya beans, fish bones (as in sardines or anchovies). |
| IRON | A key element in making new red blood cells, which carry oxygen to the muscles. | Lean red meat, liver, nuts, leafy greens like spinach, brown rice, dried apricots, beans. |
| VITAMIN D | Maintains healthy bones and teeth. | Sunshine on the skin. Oily fish, dairy, eggs, fortified breakfast cereals. |
| VITAMIN E | Protects cell membranes, meaning cells are well formed. | Leafy green vegetables, nuts and seeds, cereals, wheatgerm. |
| FOLIC ACID | Keeps the central nervous system healthy. Combined with vitamin B12, helps to build red blood cells. | Leafy green vegetables, broccoli, Brussels sprouts, peas, asparagus, chickpeas, lentils, brown rice, citrus fruit. |
| POTASSIUM | Lowers blood pressure, keeps the body's fluids in balance. | Pulses, nuts and seeds, bananas, seafood, turkey and chicken, beef, bread. |
| VITAMIN C | Maintains healthy connective tissue and cells. | Citrus fruit, berries, broccoli, Brussels sprouts, potato. |
| ZINC | Processes carbohydrates, fat, and protein. Helps make new cells and enzymes, and promotes wound healing. | Dairy, lean meat, shellfish, wheatgerm, bread. |

# A HEALTHY DIET

When planning what to eat, you need to ensure that you are getting the right quantities of nutrients necessary for good health and performance. This chart is a simple guide to how many servings per day you should have from the six main food groups.

## KEY »

**RECOMMENDED DAILY SERVINGS**
- BREAD, PASTA, AND OTHER CEREALS
- FRUIT AND VEGETABLES
- MILK AND DAIRY PRODUCTS
- MEAT, FISH, EGGS, AND OTHER SOURCES OF PROTEIN
- FOOD AND DRINKS CONTAINING FAT AND SUGAR

| 6–11 SERVINGS | 5+ SERVINGS | 2–3 SERVINGS | 2–3 SERVINGS | <1 SERVING |

# KEY FOOD GROUPS

The key to preparing for a triathlon is to follow a balanced diet that provides you with plenty of energy. Choose fresh, natural foods, such as fruit, vegetables, grains, and lean meat. Make sure you get plenty of protein (to help with muscle repair) and iron (to make red blood cells, which carry oxygen around the body). Healthy fats, found in fish, nuts, and oils, provide a good source of energy. Avoid processed foods that are high in salt, sugar, unhealthy fats, and additives. You do not need to "go on a diet" when preparing for a triathlon, but it is important to plan your meals and choose foods that will best enhance your performance.

| FOOD GROUP | ADVANTAGES | GOOD SOURCES | HOW MUCH PER DAY |
|---|---|---|---|
| WHOLEGRAINS AND STARCHES | Provide energy for muscles, reducing fatigue. Help to curb hunger, so healthy choices here can help if you want to reduce your body weight. | Wholegrain rice, pasta, bread, bagels, cereals; plain popcorn, rye crackers, stoneground wheat crackers. | Moderate amounts in the morning and afternoon. |
| FRUIT | An excellent source of vitamins, which help promote healing post-exercise. Also rich in carbohydrates and fibre. | Citrus fruit (such as oranges, limes, grapefruits, tangerines), bananas, berries, melon, kiwi. | Plenty: at least 2-4 servings. |
| VEGETABLES | Provide carbohydrates as well as vitamins and minerals, especially vitamin C, potassium, magnesium, and beta-carotene. | Salad leaves, "greens" such as broccoli, kale, and spinach, peppers (red, green, and yellow). The more variety the better. | As with fruit, eat plenty. |
| PROTEIN | Rich in amino acids, which promote muscle growth and healing. Darker meats are richer in iron and zinc. | Meat, poultry, eggs, peanut butter, tinned beans, fish, tofu. | About a fist-sized quantity of meat/tofu, plus one egg. |
| DAIRY PRODUCTS | Help maintain strong bones and reduce the risk of osteoporosis. A good source of protein, rich in calcium, vitamin D, potassium, phosphorus, and riboflavin. | Low-fat milk, cheeses, yoghurt. | 50-100g dairy or cheese, 1-2 glasses of milk. Have small, regular portions. |
| FATS AND OILS | The "good" fats are omega-3, -6 and -9. These support the immune system, nerve activity, and brain function, and help the body process vitamins. | Omega-3: oily fish, mussels; omega-6: walnut, olive, sunflower, grapeseed oils; omega-9: almonds, avocados, olives, pecans. | Moderate amounts of "healthy fats". |

# FUEL YOUR TRAINING

**Training for a triathlon** requires the right fuel, and your body will need different amounts of protein, fats, and carbohydrates depending on the intensity and duration of your training. Processed carbohydrates and sugary drinks may give you an instant boost, but they can disrupt blood-sugar levels and leave you with an insulin spike. To optimize your performance, choose foods that release energy at a slow and steady rate.

## WHAT'S THE SCORE?

The GI (glycaemic index) of these sample foods is given on a scale of 0–100, with 100 being pure sugar.

| | |
|---|---|
| • Typical energy drink | 94 |
| • Banana | 62 |
| • Wholegrain bread | 51 |
| • Brown rice | 50 |
| • Spaghetti (wholemeal) | 42 |
| • Apple | 39 |
| • Carrot | 35 |
| • Lentils | 29 |

### Q WHAT IS AN INSULIN SPIKE?

**A** When the body converts carbohydrates to glucose (a sugar used for energy), the pancreas releases the hormone insulin, which transports glucose to the body's cells. Excess glucose is stored in the muscles and liver as glycogen (see box, opposite). Foods with a low glycaemic index (GI), such as leafy greens and pulses, are broken down at a slower rate than high-GI foods, such as bread and pasta. High-GI foods can cause blood sugar levels to spike (see chart, opposite), and if there is too much glycogen for

the muscles or liver to absorb, the excess is stored as fat. High sugar levels can also result in the blood being flooded with insulin, which inhibits the use of fat for energy.

### Q HOW DO I ADAPT TO AVOID THE SPIKE?

**A** The key is to become "fat-adapted" – a process in which you train your body to use fat as fuel. You can achieve this by training for longer periods in the lower-intensity levels (see pp.160–161). You will also need to cut back on high-GI foods, and increase your intake of proteins and healthy fats (check with your

doctor before making changes to your diet). Over time, eating low-GI foods such as brown rice, quinoa, and oats will help you to become stronger, fitter, and leaner.

### Q HOW DIFFICULT IS IT?

**A** Training your body to utilize fat will take a little discipline at first, especially if you are used to a diet high in sugar and carbohydrates. Once you have become fat-adapted in the lower zones, you can slowly start to teach your body to use fat as a fuel in the higher training zones. Your stamina will improve, you will have fewer sugar

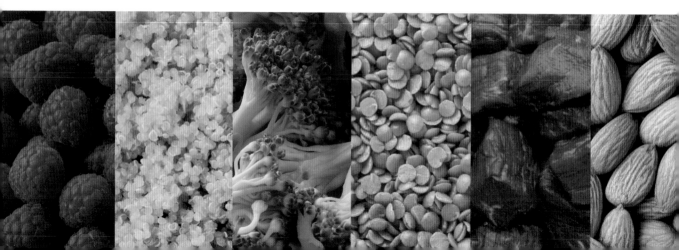

# THE GLYCAEMIC INDEX

Foods with a high glycaemic index (GI) typically give you a quick "sugar rush" followed by a crash when your energy levels dip sharply. A GI of 55 or less is considered low; 70 or more is high.

**KEY »**

◐ SLOW RELEASE
● FAST RELEASE

BLOOD GLUCOSE LEVELS

Breakfast · Mid-morning snack · Lunch · Mid-afternoon snack · Evening meal

**Time** 08:00 09:00 10:00 11:00 12:00 13:00 14:00 15:00 16:00 17:00 18:00 19:00

cravings, and you will also be far less likely to experience a hypoglycaemic crash, where your body runs out of usable energy (see panel, right).

## Q HOW MANY CALORIES DO I NEED?

**A** The average non-athlete needs 2,000 calories a day (for a female) and 2,500 (for a male). Triathletes need more than this to train efficiently and avoid illness and fatigue. Exactly how much will vary from session to session, so it is worth consulting a sports nutritionist to help you to devise a diet based on your energy requirements. It is not about eating more calories; it is about choosing the correct foods to fuel your body as you train.

## Q SHOULD I TAKE SUPPLEMENTS?

**A** The basis of any good training programme is a sensible wholefood regime (see pp.88–91). Certain vitamins, minerals, and other supplements can help provide a good back-up to a healthy diet, but they cannot replace it. Talk to your doctor or a qualified nutritionist to ensure you get the right balance for your needs.

### GLYCOGEN AND ENERGY

Carbohydrate is the primary fuel for higher-intensity training or racing. When you eat carbohydrates, any glucose that is not immediately used by the body as energy is stored in your muscles and liver as glycogen.

Most people can store around 2,000kcal of glycogen, which is enough for approximately 90 minutes of exercise. How much you can store may vary, but you can train your muscles to increase the amount they absorb.

If your glycogen stores become depleted, you may "hit the wall" – your body suddenly runs out of usable energy and you experience extreme tiredness. To prevent this, make sure you are well fuelled before the race, and if necessary boost your energy levels with sports drinks or gels.

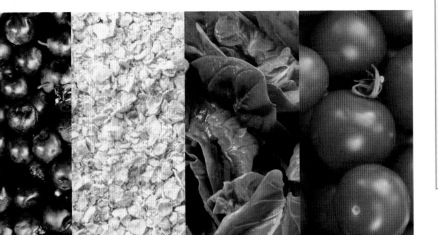

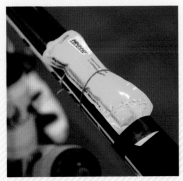

# HYDRATION FOR ATHLETES

**It is important to keep hydrated** as you train and drink whenever you are thirsty. Take a water bottle with you so that you can top up your hydration levels as and when you need. If you prefer, you can use commercial sports drinks, which are designed to help to replenish fluids at different stages of exercise.

**Q HOW DO I AVOID DEHYDRATION?**

**A** As you sweat, you lose electrolytes (essential minerals stored in the body, such as sodium, potassium, and zinc). If you start to feel thirsty, you may be becoming dehydrated, so it's a good idea to have a drink at this point. Make sure, however, that you don't over-drink as this can lead to "exercise-associated hyponatremia" (EAH) - an imbalance in electrolytes that can be fatal. Drink whenever you feel thirsty, but don't consume more water than your body needs.

## SPORTS DRINKS

There are three kinds of sports drink designed to help you rehydrate during and after exercise. Each type contains a different proportion of water, carbohydrates, and electrolytes, so check that you are drinking the right one at the right time (and factor in the calorie count when planning your day's diet). The table below is a guide to which type of drink to consume and when.

| TYPE OF DRINK | GLUCOSE | PURPOSE | WHEN BEST TO DRINK |
|---|---|---|---|
| HYPOTONIC | 2% | Quickly replenishes water lost during exercise and replaces minerals such as sodium and potassium. | In hot weather and when you are sweating a lot. Can be drunk before, during, and after a workout. |
| ISOTONIC | 4-6% | Replaces fluid and electrolytes lost during prolonged exercise sessions. Contains fructose or glucose, allowing the slow release of carbohydrates to maintain energy reserves. | During a workout or run. These drinks contain the same proportion of salt and water as your body's natural fluid balance, helping to maintain your carbohydrate–electrolyte balance during exercise. |
| HYPERTONIC | 10%+ | Supplements your daily carbohydrate intake. Provides the muscles with fuel and can be used as a recovery drink after a hard session. | After exercise. Hypertonic drinks are very high in carbohydrates and can interfere with fluid and electrolyte absorption if drunk while exercising. |

## ARE YOU DEHYDRATED?

The easiest way to check whether you are dehydrated is to collect a sample of your urine in a transparent glass and examine its colour. Ideally, your urine will be one of the first three colours shown in the chart. If it is any darker, you should rehydrate as soon as possible.

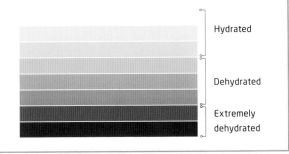

Hydrated

Dehydrated

Extremely dehydrated

## Q HOW DO I BALANCE MY ELECTROLYTES?

**A** In the days leading up to the race, you can add small amounts of sea or rock salt to your food (ask a sports nutritionist for advice). Commercial sports drinks are a useful option, or you can add about half a teaspoon of sea or rock salt to your water bottle to balance the electrolytes you will lose in sweat.

## Q WHAT SHOULD I AVOID?

**A** If you drink too much before you set off, the excess water will slosh about in your stomach. Instead, taking 3 or 4 sips from your water bottle every 15-20 minutes is probably enough: use your training sessions to see what is right for you. Pre-race nerves can make your mouth dry, causing you to sip more than you need: try swilling your mouth with water then spitting it out, and then drink as and when you need.

## Q CAN I DRINK CAFFEINE?

**A** Caffeine is a stimulant, which gives you energy; it is also a diuretic, which causes you to urinate more frequently. The ideal solution is to cut back on caffeine in the weeks leading up to a triathlon, then have a caffeinated drink during the running section - this will help to increase the stimulating effects of caffeine during the final stage of the race.

# FLUID GAIN AND LOSS

The human body takes in and excretes water in various different ways. The average percentages of fluid gain and loss are shown in the diagram below.

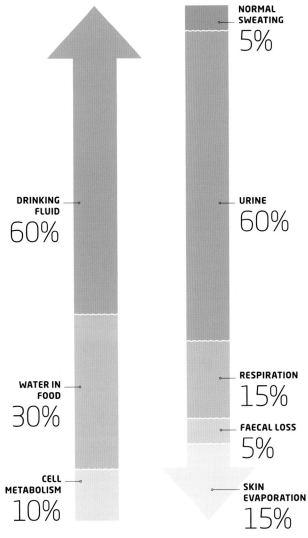

NORMAL SWEATING
5%

URINE
60%

DRINKING FLUID
60%

WATER IN FOOD
30%

CELL METABOLISM
10%

RESPIRATION
15%

FAECAL LOSS
5%

SKIN EVAPORATION
15%

**WATER INTAKE**
Your body gains fluid from three sources: drinks, the water found in food, and "metabolic water" - fluid that is released when you burn carbohydrates and fats.

**WATER LOSS**
You lose water in five main ways, though your fluid loss will vary depending on the air humidity and temperature, and the intensity and duration of your training session.

# STRENGTH AND CONDITIONING

**Strength and conditioning** is a vital part of training for all triathletes, as it improves structural support and increases your body's strength and endurance. However, it will not make you a better athlete on its own, so make sure you don't spend hours in the gym pumping iron at the expense of swim, bike, or run time. Training should be completed in three phases.

> " THERE IS **NO SPORT** YOU COULD BE **TOO STRONG** FOR. BUT **WEAKNESS** WILL CAUSE **INJURY AND INEFFICIENCY**. STRENGTH TRAINING IS ESPECIALLY IMPORTANT FOR **WOMEN AND OLDER PEOPLE**. "

## PHASE ONE FOUNDATION

Phase One prepares the body for the intense training that is to come; it should begin approximately six months before the start of the race season. Complete as many perfect repetitions as you can during the recommended time frame. This sample chart provides initial durations; increase the length of time you perform each exercise for by 10 seconds each week.

### KEY »

**SETS**
A number of repetitions separated by a short period of rest - for example, two sets of five repetitions.

**REPETITIONS/DURATION**
"Reps" are the number of times an exercise should be repeated, usually within a single set. Duration is how long an exercise should be repeated or held for.

**REST**
The suggested length of recovery period between individual sets.

**UPPER BODY**
Exercises to work the muscles of your chest, neck, shoulders, and arms - vital for directing your body's movement through the water during the swim phase.

**TRUNK**
Exercises to work the muscles from your abdomen to your pelvis. These muscles interact to stabilize your spine, providing a solid base for your legs and arms.

**LOWER BODY**
Exercises to work your hips and legs, which play an important role in all the triathlon disciplines, particularly bike and run.

**FULL BODY**
Exercises to work muscles all over your body, challenging multiple muscle groups simultaneously to build all-over strength for this endurance sport.

**» AIM OF PROGRAMME:**
STRENGTH AND ENDURANCE PREPARATION

**» DURATION OF PROGRAMME:**
2-3 TIMES PER WEEK FOR 6-12 WEEKS

| | EXERCISE | SETS | REPS/DURATION | REST |
|---|---|---|---|---|
| 01 | STANDING PAUSING WITH ANKLE WEIGHTS | 1 x | 60 SECS EACH SIDE | 30 SECS |
| 02 | STANDING BALANCE WITH EYES CLOSED | 1 x | 60 SECS EACH SIDE | 30 SECS |
| 03 | BACK BRIDGE | 1 x | 60 SECS | 30 SECS |
| 04 | SINGLE-LEG BRIDGE | 1 x | 30 SECS EACH SIDE | 30 SECS |
| 05 | SIDE PLANK | 1 x | 30 SECS EACH SIDE | 30 SECS |
| 06 | FRONT PLANK | 1 x | 60 SECS | 30 SECS |
| 07 | SINGLE-LEG ROMANIAN DEAD LIFT | 1 x | 30 SECS EACH SIDE | 30 SECS |
| 08 | CLAM | 1 x | 60 SECS EACH SIDE | 30 SECS |
| 09 | SHOULDER ROTATION | 1 x | 60 SECS | 30 SECS |
| 10 | INTERNAL ROTATION | 1 x | 30 SECS EACH SIDE | 30 SECS |
| 11 | EXTERNAL ROTATION | 1 x | 30 SECS EACH SIDE | 30 SECS |
| 12 | BASIC SIT-UP | 1 x | 30 SECS | 30 SECS |
| 13 | BIRD DOG | 1 x | 60 SECS | 30 SECS |

# 01 **STANDING** PAUSING WITH ANKLE WEIGHTS

The three triathlon sports work your hips and ankles in a forwards-backwards motion, so working on adduction (moving your limb away from your body) and abduction (moving it towards your body) aids stability and balance.

**PROGRESSION**

**Standing flowing with ankle weights**
This progression will further improve your balance. Perform the exercise as for Standing pausing with ankle weights, but this time keep your leg moving in a continuous, flowing motion from one side to the other.

Focus on a fixed point to aid balance

1 Attach an ankle weight to your left leg. Stand in an upright position with your hands on your hips and your legs hip-distance apart. Raise your left leg out to the side. Hold for 2-3 seconds.

Raise your leg up to around 45 degrees from centre

2 Slowly and under control, move your leg across your body and slightly out to the other side. Hold for 2-3 seconds before returning your leg to the ground. Repeat the exercise, holding for 2-3 seconds in each leg position, for a total of 60 seconds. Change the ankle weight to your right leg and repeat on that side.

Control the leg movement carefully

# 02 **STANDING** BALANCE WITH EYES CLOSED

This exercise works to improve your stability, balance, and proprioception (your sense of where the parts of your body are in relation to one another) in a weight-bearing position.

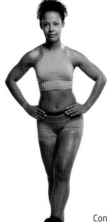

1 Attach an ankle weight to your left leg. Stand in an upright position with your legs hip-distance apart. Close your eyes.

Raise your arms out to the sides to aid balance

2 Raise your left knee towards hip-height, hinging your lower leg down towards the floor. Hold the position for 60 seconds, return to the start, and repeat with your right leg.

Engage your trunk

Centre your body weight through your right leg

# 03 **BACK** BRIDGE

This important trunk-stabilizing movement activates the large gluteal muscles in your buttocks. Use your hands to check that your hamstrings are relaxed; the effort should come from your glutes rather than your legs.

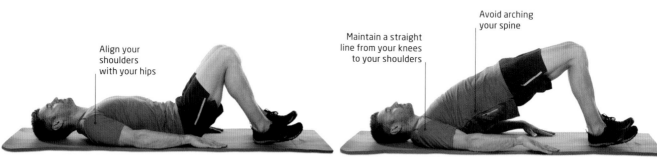

Align your shoulders with your hips

Maintain a straight line from your knees to your shoulders

Avoid arching your spine

1 Lie flat on your back with your knees bent up at an angle and your heels on the floor, hip-width apart. Place your arms at your sides, with your hands palms-down.

2 Engage your trunk. Slowly lift your buttocks off the floor until your body is in a straight line from your knees to your shoulders. Pause, then slowly reverse the movement to return to the start position. Repeat the exercise for 60 seconds.

# 04 **SINGLE-LEG** BRIDGE

Performing the bridge on one leg forces you to control the rotation and tilt of your pelvis. Ensure that you keep your hips level throughout, and avoid arching your spine.

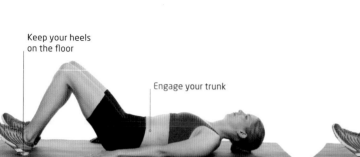

Keep your heels on the floor

Engage your trunk

Hold your thighs at a 90-degree angle to each other

Hold your body in a straight line from left knee to shoulder

1 Lie flat on your back with your feet hip-width apart and your knees at an angle. Place your hands palms-down by your sides and raise your right knee towards your chest, until your thighs are at a 90-degree angle to each other.

2 Engage your glutes and lift your buttocks off the floor until your hips are fully extended. Pause, then slowly reverse to the start position. Repeat the exercise for 30 seconds before switching to the other side.

# ⚫ 05 **SIDE** PLANK

This exercise strengthens your trunk, as well as the stabilizing muscles of your spine, lower back, and glutes – all of which are vital for the triathlon sports. Maintaining good form throughout the exercise is crucial to working your trunk in the correct way.

**PROGRESSION**

As you lift your hips into the plank position, raise your left arm and leg until you make a star shape, keeping your spine straight. Hold, then return to the start position and repeat on the other side. Raising your arm and leg will improve trunk stability, as you work harder to maintain balance.

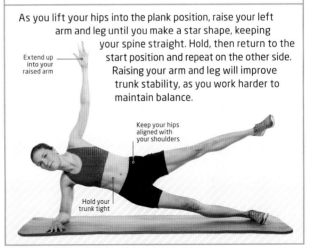

Extend up into your raised arm

Keep your hips aligned with your shoulders

Hold your trunk tight

Ensure your hips are aligned with one another and do not drop back

Avoid letting your upper shoulder drop forwards

1 Lying on your right side, prop yourself up on your right forearm. Extend your legs and keep your feet together. Make sure that your right elbow is directly under your shoulder and in line with your hips. Put your left hand on your hip.

Avoid letting your upper shoulder drop forwards

Keep your feet aligned

Keep your trunk tight and your hips lifted

2 Push downwards through your right elbow to raise your hips off the ground, making sure that you keep the ribcage elevated and your shoulders in line with each other. Keep your spine straight and your neck aligned. Hold the position for 30 seconds, taking controlled breaths and keeping your trunk engaged.

Keep your trunk engaged

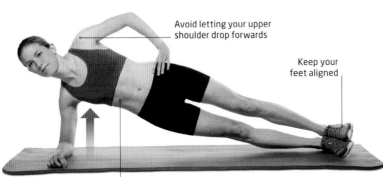

3 Slowly reverse the movement to return to the start position, then repeat on your left side. Make sure you hold the position for the same length of time on both sides of your body, to ensure that you strengthen both sides equally.

# ◐ 06 **FRONT** PLANK

Performing a front plank strengthens your transverse abdominis, the deepest of the abdominal muscles, which will provide vital trunk support during all of the triathlon stages.

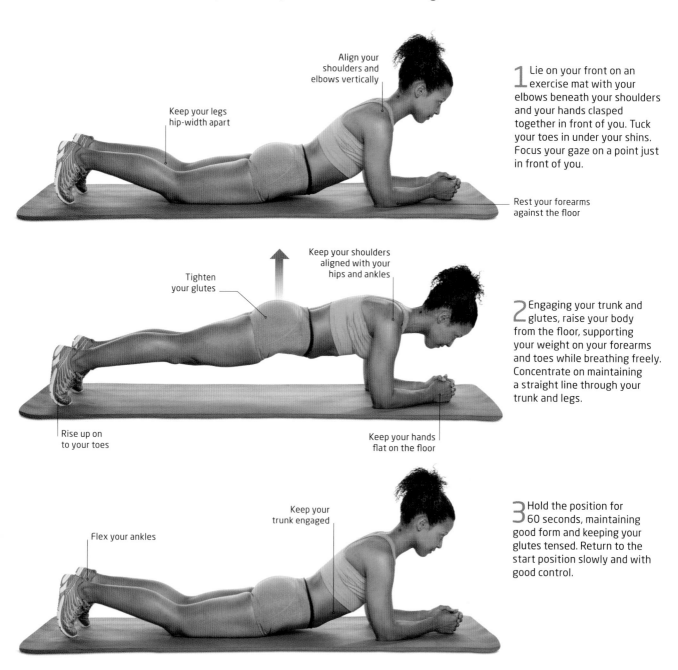

Align your shoulders and elbows vertically

Keep your legs hip-width apart

**1** Lie on your front on an exercise mat with your elbows beneath your shoulders and your hands clasped together in front of you. Tuck your toes in under your shins. Focus your gaze on a point just in front of you.

Rest your forearms against the floor

Keep your shoulders aligned with your hips and ankles

Tighten your glutes

**2** Engaging your trunk and glutes, raise your body from the floor, supporting your weight on your forearms and toes while breathing freely. Concentrate on maintaining a straight line through your trunk and legs.

Rise up on to your toes

Keep your hands flat on the floor

Keep your trunk engaged

Flex your ankles

**3** Hold the position for 60 seconds, maintaining good form and keeping your glutes tensed. Return to the start position slowly and with good control.

# 07 SINGLE-LEG ROMANIAN DEAD LIFT

This exercise strengthens your hamstrings, the key muscles you use for running. Start with dumbbells; once you've mastered this, add greater resistance by using a barbell.

> **WARNING!**
>
> Correct lifting technique is essential in this movement. Never lift with your spine bent: not only will the exercise be ineffective, but you will also risk spinal injury. Practise with light weights until perfect, and if possible spend time with a qualified lifting coach.

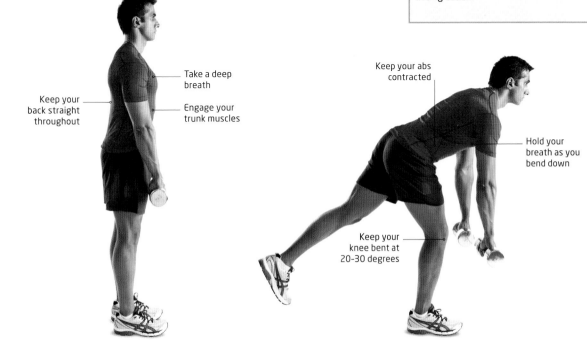

Take a deep breath

Keep your back straight throughout

Engage your trunk muscles

Keep your abs contracted

Hold your breath as you bend down

Keep your knee bent at 20-30 degrees

**1** Stand with your feet hip-width apart and position your right foot about half a step in front of your left foot. Hold a dumbbell in each hand, using an overhand grip (see p.108).

**2** Bend from your waist and push your hips backwards to lower the dumbbells towards your right foot. Bend your right leg and lift your left leg behind you for balance.

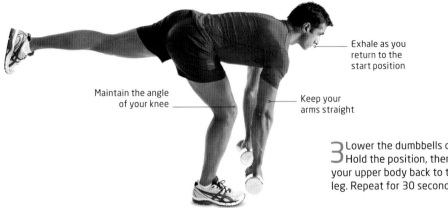

Maintain the angle of your knee

Keep your arms straight

Exhale as you return to the start position

**3** Lower the dumbbells down your shin as far as you can. Hold the position, then push your hips forwards to bring your upper body back to the start position and lower your leg. Repeat for 30 seconds before switching to the other side.

# 08 CLAM

This simple exercise strengthens your medial glutes, which are muscles used constantly in triathlon, especially for stabilizing your hips and knees. It's an endurance muscle, so work it for longer periods or more reps to feel the benefit.

## RESISTANCE BANDS

Adding a band around your knees forces your muscles to work harder; once you can complete three minutes, use a thicker band for more resistance. If at first you find this exercise too difficult, begin without bands.

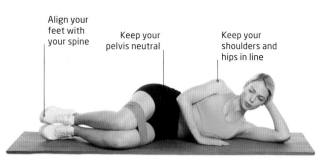

Align your feet with your spine

Keep your pelvis neutral

Keep your shoulders and hips in line

Ensure you keep your feet stacked

Keep your hips forwards and aligned one above the other

1 Put a resistance band around your thighs and lie on your left side, bending both your hips and knees at a 90-degree angle. Lean your head on your left arm. Bend your right arm at the elbow and place your right hand on to the floor in front of you.

2 Engage your trunk and lift the knee of your right leg, rotating at your hip. Lift your knee as far as it will go without straining, before slowly lowering it back to the start position. Repeat for 60 seconds before switching to the other side.

# 09 SHOULDER ROTATION

This exercise is designed to increase the strength and endurance of the deltoids (main shoulder muscles), vital for your swim stroke.

## PROGRESSION

To make this exercise harder, increase the duration (see p.94), or add wrist weights to both arms.

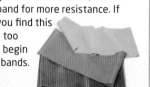

Rotate your arms from your shoulder

Stand in an upright position with your legs slightly wider than hip-width apart, and your arms held straight out at shoulder height. Start rotating your hands in circles the size of a golf ball. After 20 seconds, increase the size of the rotations to that of a tennis ball. After a further 20 seconds, increase to the size of a football.

Maintain your arm height; don't slump your shoulders

# 10 INTERNAL ROTATION

This exercise strengthens the smaller muscles of the shoulder girdle - the rotator cuff muscles - which help keep your shoulders stable during front crawl.

Keep your head up and look forwards

Put your left hand on your hip

Keep your legs braced throughout exercise

1 Stand sideways to a pulley set at about waist height. Hold the handle securely with your right hand, and grip a bottle or folded towel between your arm and chest to help you maintain the correct position. Bend your elbow to 90 degrees and turn your arm out away from your body.

2 Keep your shoulders, hips, and feet in line. Pull the handle slowly and under control towards the middle of your body. Keep your elbow tight in to your side.

3 Bring your lower arm across as far as is comfortable, maintaining a right angle at your elbow. Return slowly to the start position. Repeat for 30 seconds before switching to the other side.

# 11 EXTERNAL ROTATION

This simple pulley exercise continues on from internal rotation (above) to work your shoulder muscles away from your body, rather than towards it.

Keep your head up and look straight ahead

Keep your shoulders level

Encircle the handle with your thumb

1 Stand sideways to a pulley set at about waist height. Reach across your body and grip the handle with your right hand. Grip a bottle or folded towel between your arm and chest. Keep your shoulders, hips, and feet in line, and your legs braced throughout the exercise. Hold the frame for support, if necessary.

2 With your elbow bent and tight to your body, move your lower arm across and away from your body. When you reach your full range of movement, return to the start position under control. Repeat for 30 seconds before switching to the other side.

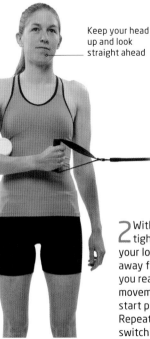

# 12 **BASIC** SIT-UP

The sit-up is an effective exercise for strengthening your abdominals and increasing hip flexion. Focus on using your trunk to drive the movement, and avoid straining your neck.

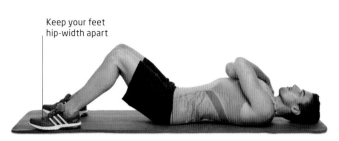

Keep your feet hip-width apart

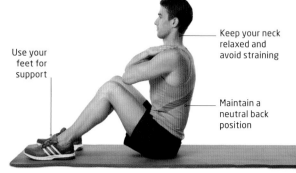

Use your feet for support

Keep your neck relaxed and avoid straining

Maintain a neutral back position

**1** Lie on your back with your feet on the floor and your knees bent. Cross your arms across your chest. Engage your trunk muscles and raise your torso upwards, leaving just your buttocks and feet on the floor.

**2** Pause at the edge of the movement, then slowly lower your upper body to the start position, controlling the movement with your trunk. Repeat the exercise for 30 seconds.

# 13 **BIRD** DOG

This exercise relies on your trunk muscles to keep you stable; it also strengthens the muscles along the back of your body (glutes and erector spinae).

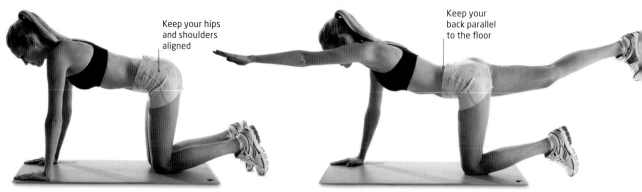

Keep your hips and shoulders aligned

Keep your back parallel to the floor

**1** Kneel on all fours, with your knees directly below your hips and your hands positioned below your shoulders, pressed flat on the floor with your fingers pointing forwards. Keep your spine in a neutral position and align your head with your back. Engage your trunk.

**2** Raise your left arm straight in front of you, palm-down. Stretch out your right leg and raise it behind you until it is parallel to the floor, using your trunk to keep your body stable. Hold briefly, then return your arm and leg to the floor. Repeat on alternating sides for 60 seconds.

## PHASE TWO WINTER

During this phase you will focus on training with greater loads and at a higher intensity, targeting the major muscles groups for triathlon: your trunk's latissimi dorsi, and your glutes, quads, and hamstrings. Aim to either increase the length of time you perform each exercise for by 10 seconds each week or to increase the number of reps.

**» AIM OF PROGRAMME:**
INCREASING STRENGTH AND ENDURANCE

**» DURATION OF PROGRAMME:**
2-3 TIMES PER WEEK FOR 6-12 WEEKS

| | EXERCISE | SETS | REPS/DURATION | REST |
|---|---|---|---|---|
| 14 | ADDUCTION | 1 x | 90 SECS | 30 SECS |
| 15 | ON ALL 4'S ALPHABET | 1 x | 1 REP EACH SIDE | 30 SECS |
| 16 | NORDIC HAMMIES | 1-3 x | 8 REPS | 1 MIN |
| 17 | PRESS-UP | 1-3 x | 8 REPS | 1 MIN |
| 18 | FRONT PLANK ROTATION | 1 x | 60 SECS | 30 SECS |
| 19 | BALLISTIC SIT-UP | 1-3 x | 8 REPS | 30 SECS |
| 20 | BASIC CLEAN AND JERK | 1-3 x | 8 REPS | 1 MIN |
| 21 | CHIN-UP | 1-3 x | 8 REPS | 1 MIN |

# 14 ADDUCTION

Adduction works on the stabilizing muscles of the inside of your leg, as well as the antagonist muscles on the outside of your opposite leg. Strengthening these will aid stability during running and improve knee alignment for cycling.

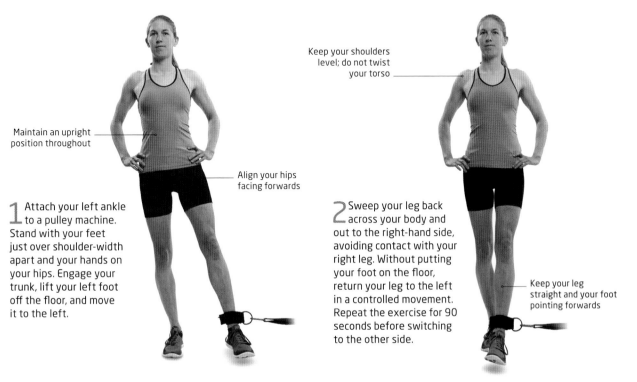

Keep your shoulders level; do not twist your torso

Maintain an upright position throughout

Align your hips facing forwards

Keep your leg straight and your foot pointing forwards

1 Attach your left ankle to a pulley machine. Stand with your feet just over shoulder-width apart and your hands on your hips. Engage your trunk, lift your left foot off the floor, and move it to the left.

2 Sweep your leg back across your body and out to the right-hand side, avoiding contact with your right leg. Without putting your foot on the floor, return your leg to the left in a controlled movement. Repeat the exercise for 90 seconds before switching to the other side.

# 15 ON ALL 4'S ALPHABET

This exercise builds on Bird dog (p.102), adding more challenge to trunk control with new hand and leg movements.

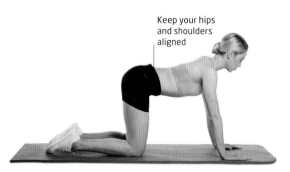

Keep your hips and shoulders aligned

**1** Kneel on all fours, with your knees below your hips and your hands below your shoulders, pressed flat on the floor with your fingers pointing forwards. Keep your spine in a neutral position. Engage your trunk.

Trace each letter with your foot, keeping your leg straight

Move your whole leg from the hip

**2** Raise your left arm straight in front of you, palm-down. Stretch your right leg out behind you, using your trunk to keep you stable. Draw each letter of the alphabet in the air using your right foot, moving your leg with it. Return to the start position and repeat on the other side.

## PROGRESSION

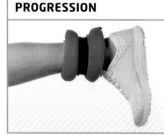

**As you become stronger**, try drawing the alphabet with your hand and foot simultaneously. Once you've mastered this, try adding an ankle weight.

# 16 NORDIC HAMMIES

Great for strengthening your hamstrings for running and cycling, this exercise requires the assistance of a partner before attempting it alone. Good form is key.

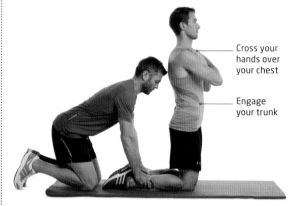

Cross your hands over your chest

Engage your trunk

**1** Kneel down on a mat, with a partner holding down (but not sitting on) your ankles. Ensure that your body is aligned straight up from your knees to your shoulders.

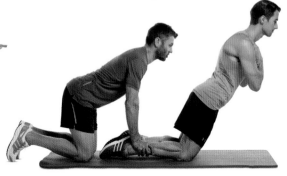

**2** Engage your abdominals and lean forwards as far as you can, using your hamstrings to control the motion. Contract your hamstrings to raise yourself back to an upright position.

## TIP

**If you are doing this exercise on your own**, hook your ankles under a bench or bar.

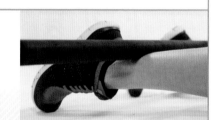

# 17 PRESS-UP (FEET)

This is one of the simplest but most effective exercises for developing strength in your shoulders, arms, chest, and trunk. Its added benefit is that it requires no apparatus to practise. Maintain good form throughout.

1 Lie face-down on the floor with your hands under and a little wider than your shoulders. Coming up on to your toes, raise your body up off the floor, with your arms straight and your fingers extended. Keep your legs, upper body, and head in a straight line throughout.

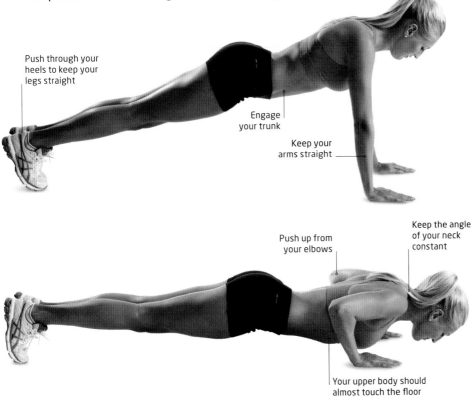

Push through your heels to keep your legs straight

Engage your trunk

Keep your arms straight

2 Pause at the top of the movement, then lower your body slowly and under control until your upper body almost touches the floor. Hold the position briefly, then push your upper body up from your elbows until your arms are straight. Maintain a neutral spine throughout.

Push up from your elbows

Keep the angle of your neck constant

Your upper body should almost touch the floor

## VARIATION: PRESS-UP (KNEES)

1 If you find the Press-Up above too hard at first, support your body weight on your knees, with your arms straight and hands a little wider than your shoulders.

2 Lower your body slowly and under control until your upper body almost touches the floor. Hold briefly, then push up from your elbows until you are back in the start position.

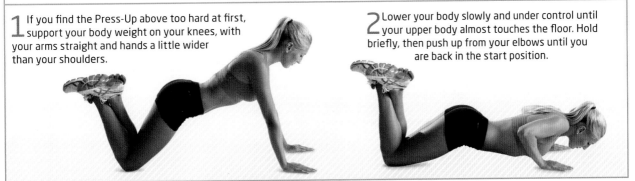

# 18 FRONT PLANK ROTATION

A progression from the front (p.98) and side plank (p.97), this exercise adds in a rotation to further strengthen your trunk. This is a great strengthening exercise for all three disciplines.

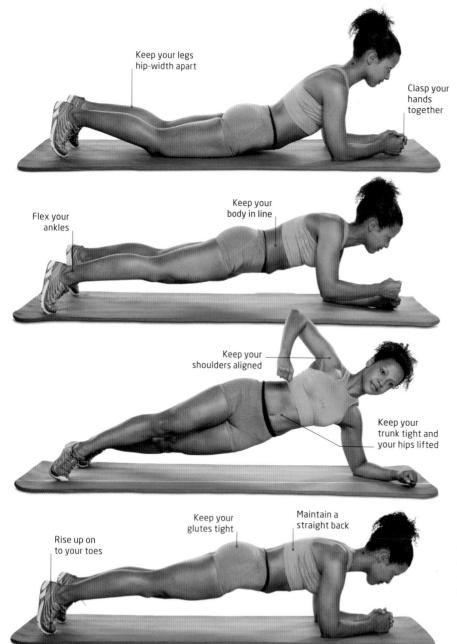

Keep your legs hip-width apart

Clasp your hands together

1 Lie face-down with your elbows beneath your shoulders, your forearms resting on the floor, and your hands together.

Flex your ankles

Keep your body in line

2 Engage your trunk and glutes, and raise your body off the floor, supporting your weight on your forearms and toes. Breathe calmly and focus on maintaining good form, holding a straight line through your trunk and legs. Keeping your hips aligned, raise your right elbow slightly off the floor.

Keep your shoulders aligned

Keep your trunk tight and your hips lifted

3 Supporting your body weight on your left forearm and toes, push off the floor, rotating through your hips and shoulders, until your body is facing outwards to your right. Place your right hand on your hip and hold the position for one minute.

Rise up on to your toes

Keep your glutes tight

Maintain a straight back

4 Reverse the rotational movement slowly and with control to return first to the plank position, and then to the starting position. Repeat on the other side.

# 19 BALLISTIC SIT-UP

A little more demanding than the basic sit-up, this dynamic exercise strengthens the muscles used in the extension and catch phases of swim (see pp.16–17).

**TIP**

**If you don't have a partner** to do this exercise with, throw the ball against a wall instead, catching it as it bounces back.

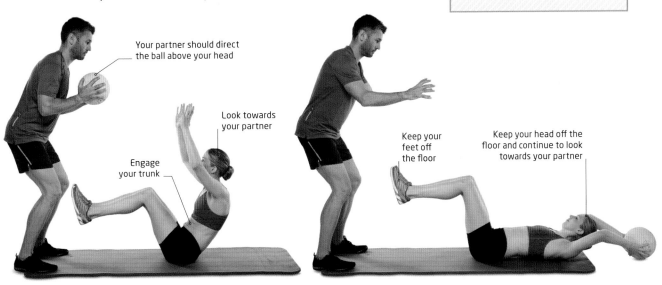

Your partner should direct the ball above your head

Look towards your partner

Engage your trunk

Keep your feet off the floor

Keep your head off the floor and continue to look towards your partner

1 Sit up straight, with your feet off the floor, legs bent at right angles, and your arms stretched. Roll backwards, and as you do so get your partner to throw you a medicine ball. Reach above your head to catch it with both hands.

2 Using the momentum of the ball, keep rolling backwards until your back touches the floor. Extend your arms behind your head until the ball touches the ground. Pause briefly.

**VARIATION: V SIT-UP**

Lie down with your arms stretched behind your head and your feet together. Engage your trunk and crunch up with your upper body, simultaneously bringing your arms over in front of you and your legs towards your chest as far as you can. Pause before unfolding under control back to the start position.

Keep your hands relaxed and do not strain your neck

Keep your knees together

Engage your trunk

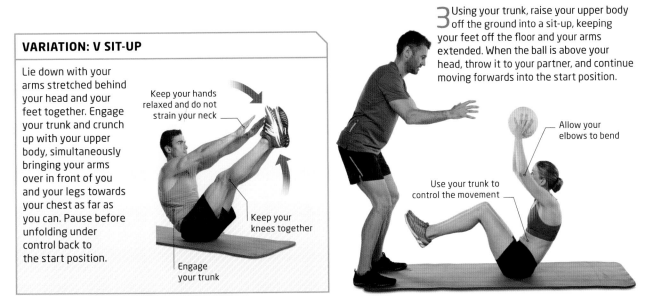

3 Using your trunk, raise your upper body off the ground into a sit-up, keeping your feet off the floor and your arms extended. When the ball is above your head, throw it to your partner, and continue moving forwards into the start position.

Allow your elbows to bend

Use your trunk to control the movement

# ⓘ 20 **BASIC** CLEAN AND JERK

This explosive exercise is technically difficult, but great for building strength and stability. This version includes a brief pause between the "clean" (the lift to your chest) and "jerk" (the above-head raise) movements to make it safer and easier.

## WARNING

Carry out all lifts in a safe and controlled environment. This complex movement demands excellent technique, balance, and co-ordination. Practise with light weights until perfect, and if possible spend time with a qualified lifting coach. Start with weights of around 15 per cent of your body weight, and increase by 10 per cent each week. Always ensure that your body is in the correct alignment before attempting a lift. Your back should be flat and your shoulders must be directly above the bar.

## HAND AND FOOT POSITIONING

Correct positioning is key to safe lifting technique; always check these details before attempting a lift.

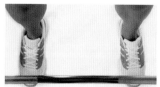

**Foot position**
Position your feet slightly wider than hip-width apart, with your toes just visible in front of the bar.

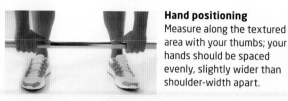

**Hand positioning**
Measure along the textured area with your thumbs; your hands should be spaced evenly, slightly wider than shoulder-width apart.

**Grip**
Curl your fingers around the bar and tuck your thumbs over the top of your fingers.

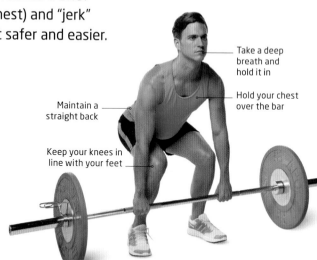

Take a deep breath and hold it in

Hold your chest over the bar

Maintain a straight back

Keep your knees in line with your feet

1 Squat with your feet hip-width apart, your back straight, and your buttocks as low as possible. Grip the barbell. Apply tension to the bar, feeling the weight coming through your glutes and quads – not your lower back – and down through your heels.

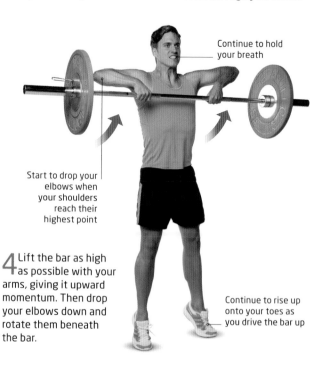

Continue to hold your breath

Start to drop your elbows when your shoulders reach their highest point

4 Lift the bar as high as possible with your arms, giving it upward momentum. Then drop your elbows down and rotate them beneath the bar.

Continue to rise up onto your toes as you drive the bar up

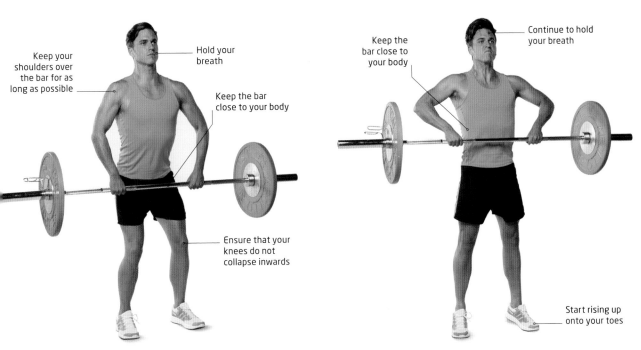

Keep your shoulders over the bar for as long as possible

Hold your breath

Keep the bar close to your body

Ensure that your knees do not collapse inwards

Keep the bar close to your body

Continue to hold your breath

Start rising up onto your toes

2 Drive the bar upwards, using your glutes and quads to power the movement and give the weight momentum. Keep your arms straight until the bar comes past your knees, then bend at the elbows.

3 Forcefully extend your hips, knees, and ankles, keeping the bar close to your body. Shrug your shoulders upwards hard, lifting the bar with your arms and bending your elbows out to the sides.

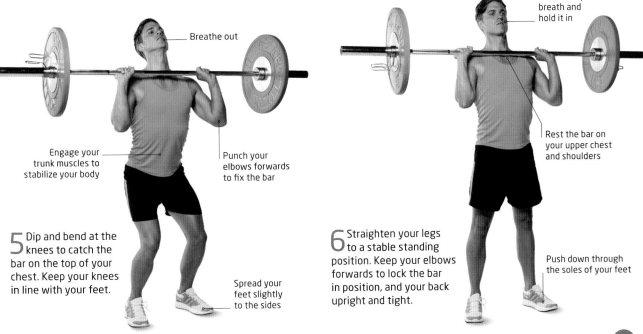

Breathe out

Engage your trunk muscles to stabilize your body

Punch your elbows forwards to fix the bar

Spread your feet slightly to the sides

Take a deep breath and hold it in

Rest the bar on your upper chest and shoulders

Push down through the soles of your feet

5 Dip and bend at the knees to catch the bar on the top of your chest. Keep your knees in line with your feet.

6 Straighten your legs to a stable standing position. Keep your elbows forwards to lock the bar in position, and your back upright and tight.

See over for steps 7-10 »

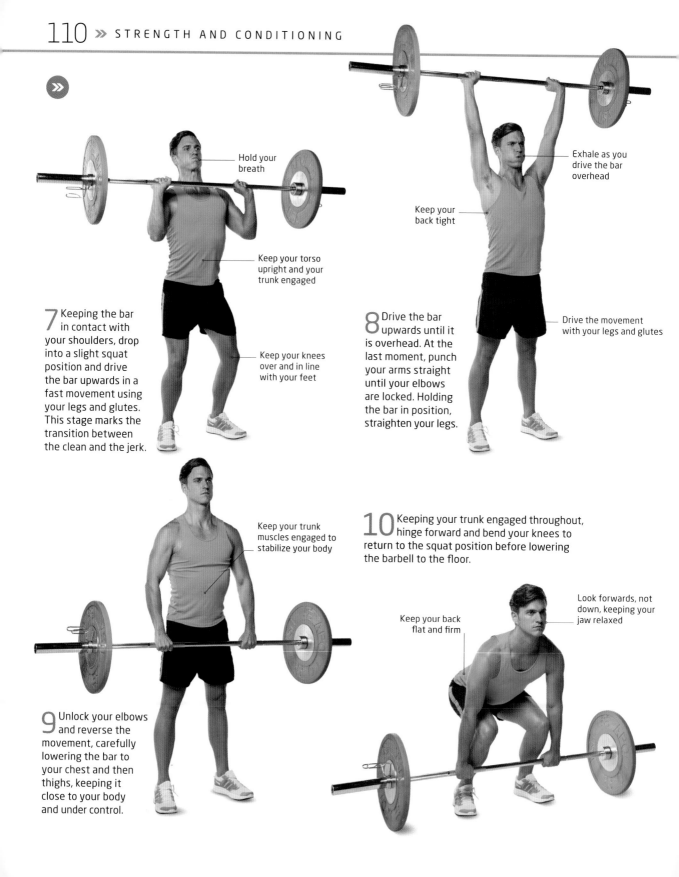

Hold your breath

Keep your torso upright and your trunk engaged

Keep your knees over and in line with your feet

**7** Keeping the bar in contact with your shoulders, drop into a slight squat position and drive the bar upwards in a fast movement using your legs and glutes. This stage marks the transition between the clean and the jerk.

Exhale as you drive the bar overhead

Keep your back tight

Drive the movement with your legs and glutes

**8** Drive the bar upwards until it is overhead. At the last moment, punch your arms straight until your elbows are locked. Holding the bar in position, straighten your legs.

Keep your trunk muscles engaged to stabilize your body

**9** Unlock your elbows and reverse the movement, carefully lowering the bar to your chest and then thighs, keeping it close to your body and under control.

**10** Keeping your trunk engaged throughout, hinge forward and bend your knees to return to the squat position before lowering the barbell to the floor.

Look forwards, not down, keeping your jaw relaxed

Keep your back flat and firm

# 21 CHIN-UP

This exercise is one of the most effective strength builders
for the latissimus dorsi – the muscles in your back used during
the catch and pull phases when you swim (see pp.12-13).

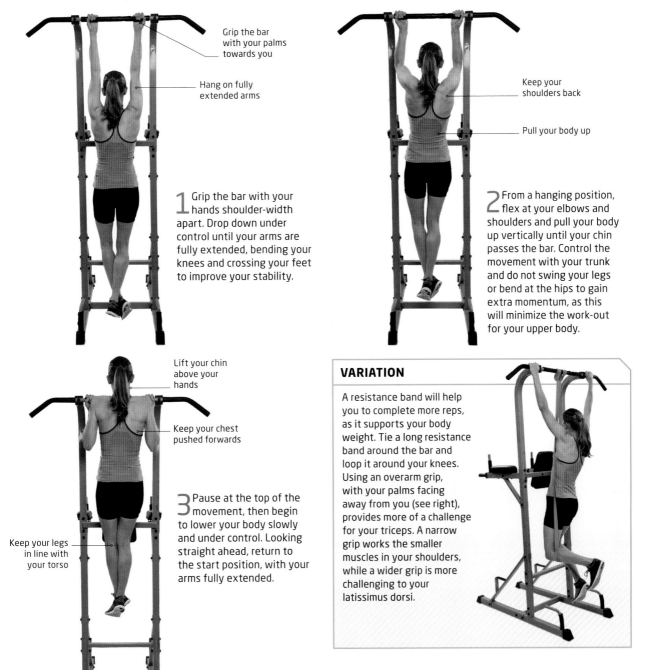

Grip the bar
with your palms
towards you

Hang on fully
extended arms

**1** Grip the bar with your
hands shoulder-width
apart. Drop down under
control until your arms are
fully extended, bending your
knees and crossing your feet
to improve your stability.

Keep your
shoulders back

Pull your body up

**2** From a hanging position,
flex at your elbows and
shoulders and pull your body
up vertically until your chin
passes the bar. Control the
movement with your trunk
and do not swing your legs
or bend at the hips to gain
extra momentum, as this
will minimize the work-out
for your upper body.

Lift your chin
above your
hands

Keep your chest
pushed forwards

Keep your legs
in line with
your torso

**3** Pause at the top of the
movement, then begin
to lower your body slowly
and under control. Looking
straight ahead, return to
the start position, with your
arms fully extended.

## VARIATION

A resistance band will help
you to complete more reps,
as it supports your body
weight. Tie a long resistance
band around the bar and
loop it around your knees.
Using an overarm grip,
with your palms facing
away from you (see right),
provides more of a challenge
for your triceps. A narrow
grip works the smaller
muscles in your shoulders,
while a wider grip is more
challenging to your
latissimus dorsi.

## PHASE THREE PREPARATION

By the time you start phase three, your body will be much stronger and you will be able to complete higher intensity swim, bike, and run sessions. Phase three will help you to maintain your strength levels and prepare for racing. Assess your performance, and aim to focus on any remaining weaknesses in your training.

» **AIM OF PROGRAMME:** PREPARING FOR RACING, MAINTAINING STRENGTH, ADDRESSING WEAKNESSES

» **DURATION OF PROGRAMME:** 2-3 TIMES PER WEEK FOR 6-12 WEEKS

| | EXERCISE | SETS | REPS/DURATION | REST |
|---|---|---|---|---|
| 20 | BASIC CLEAN AND JERK (pp.108-110) | 1-3 x | 12 REPS | 3 MINS |
| 21 | CHIN-UP WITH BAND (p.111) | 1 x | 30 REPS | 3 MINS |
| 19 | BALLISTIC SIT-UP (p.107) | 1 x | 30 REPS | 90 SECS |
| 22 | SINGLE-LEG JUMP SQUAT | 1 x | 30 REPS EACH SIDE | 3 MINS |
| 02 | STANDING BALANCE WITH EYES CLOSED (p.95) | 1 x | 60 SECS EACH SIDE | 30 SECS |
| 23 | NORDIC HAMMIES INTO BALLISTIC PRESS-UP | 1 x | 30 REPS | 3 MINS |
| 24 | SUPERMAN BENCH RAISE | 1 x | 15 REPS | 3 MINS |

## ◖ 22 SINGLE-LEG JUMP SQUAT

This exercise addresses imbalance by working on each leg individually. Once you have perfected this exercise, add light weights to work on strength as well as endurance.

" THINK: DO I NEED TO BE **STRONGER** OR DO I NEED TO IMPROVE MY **ENDURANCE**? "

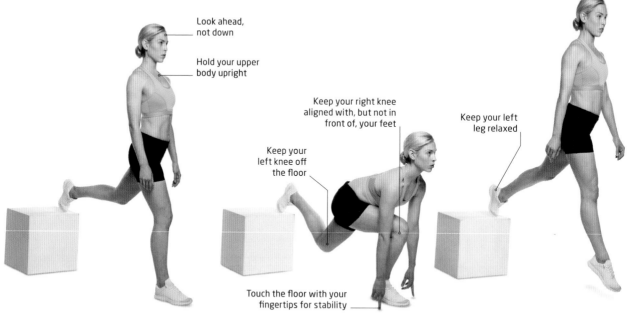

Look ahead, not down

Hold your upper body upright

Keep your right knee aligned with, but not in front of, your feet

Keep your left knee off the floor

Keep your left leg relaxed

Touch the floor with your fingertips for stability

1 Stand with your back to a knee-high bench or similar, and bend your left leg back to rest on it. Hold your arms loosely at your sides.

2 Take a deep breath, then bend your right knee into a deep lunge using your glutes, quads, and hamstrings. Bend your upper body forwards from the waist, keeping your back straight. Pause when your right thigh is parallel to the floor.

3 Raise yourself back up using your right leg. As you reach an upright position, breathe out and spring into a small jump using your right leg. Lower yourself back into the lunge and complete 30 reps before switching sides.

# 🔘 23 **NORDIC HAMMIES**
## INTO BALLISTIC PRESS-UP

As with Nordic hammies (p.104), you can do this with a partner or by hooking your ankles under a bar. Complete the exercise with a partner first, so that they can check your body position.

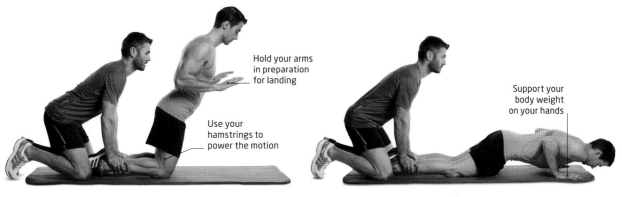

Hold your arms in preparation for landing

Use your hamstrings to power the motion

Support your body weight on your hands

**1** Kneel upright on a mat, with a partner holding on to your ankles to stabilize your legs. Ensure that your body is aligned from your knees to your shoulders. Engage your hamstrings and abdominals and lean forwards as far as you can.

**2** Use your hamstrings to control the movement of your body as far as you can, before using your hands to support your body weight in a press-up position. Press-up back to an upright position, driving the movement by contracting your hamstrings and engaging your trunk.

# 🔘 24 **SUPERMAN** BENCH RAISE

A progression from Bird dog (p.102) and On all 4's alphabet (p.104), this exercise adds an extra element of stability to further strengthen your trunk.

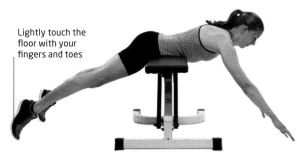

Lightly touch the floor with your fingers and toes

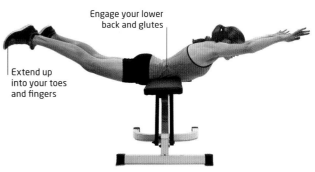

Engage your lower back and glutes

Extend up into your toes and fingers

**1** Lie face-down across a bench, so that your weight is evenly balanced. Space your legs hip-width apart and spread your hands out wide in front of you.

**2** Engaging your trunk, slowly raise your arms and legs off the ground and up into the air. Hold in position for 2-3 seconds. Slowly lower yourself to the start position, just brushing your fingers and toes on the floor before repeating.

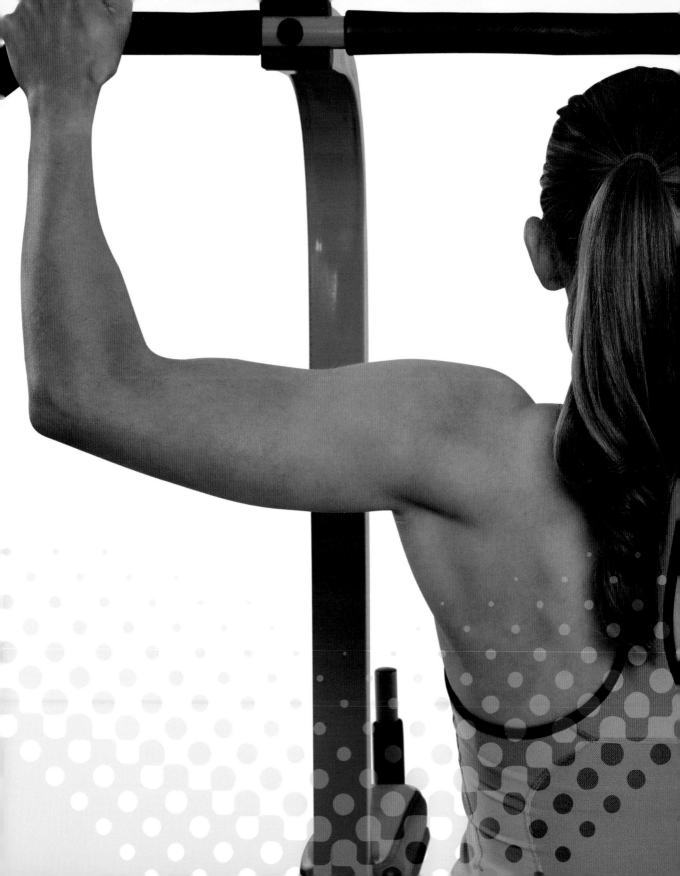

# PERSONALIZE YOUR TRAINING

# GOOD TRAINING PRINCIPLES

**The five Ps** - "Planning and Preparation Prevent Poor Performance" - are particularly apt for triathlon. When it comes to preparing your body for the challenge of a triathlon, the planning phase is most important. Building your training plan around a few basic principles will establish a solid foundation from which you can race towards your goals.

**10**%

THE GUIDELINE PERCENTAGE BY WHICH YOU SHOULD INCREASE YOUR EXERCISE HOURS/ DISTANCES PER WEEK

## YOUR ROUTE TO SUCCESS

### BE DEDICATED

Dedication is vital. Anyone can exercise when they're cheerful and the sun's out, but the days when you don't feel like it are key to mental toughness and success. There may be days, or weeks, when you're not well or you're injured, so make the most of every day that you do get out and train.

### BE SPECIFIC

If you want to master the technical elements of swimming, swim more. If you want to get better at cycling uphill, cycle uphill more. If you want to run faster, run more. This is called specificity: no amount of pumping iron or doing sit-ups will make you a better swimmer, cyclist, or runner. Make sure you train for what the triathlon will demand of you.

### PROGRESS GRADUALLY

Be sensible and build your training up slowly. Jumping from a 30-minute run to running 90 minutes is likely to result in injury and set back your entire training programme. Similarly, you'll be more vulnerable to illness if you exhaust yourself by suddenly doubling your weekly training hours, say from 10 to 20. Ideally, increase your training volume by about 10 per cent per week. If you take care of yourself and follow this rule, you'll progress more in the long term.

# COMPONENTS OF A TRAINING SESSION

For an easy swim, bike, or run, gradually building up the pace may suffice. However, at Level 3 or above you need to include a variety of stages to get the maximum benefits and reduce the risk of injury. Follow this four-stage process in your training sessions to get the most out of your programme.

### WARM UP

Beginning at a low intensity lubricates the joints with synovial fluid, reducing wear. It also raises your heart rate, increasing blood flow to the muscles (see pp.160-161).

### PRE-MAIN

Once warmed up, do specific drills relating to the discipline that you're training for, or you might want to do some shorter sprints above the pace of the main set, to prepare.

### MAIN SET

This is designed to work on your current goals, or perhaps your weaknesses. You can be specific as you approach a race, for example by prepping for a particular course.

### COOL DOWN

The body returns to normal after exertion. Post swim you may want to do a few easy laps; on the bike ease off slightly for 10 minutes; after running try flushing exercises (pp.74-75).

### USE IT OR LOSE IT

Fitness is a reversible achievement: any improvements you make as a result of training will start to go away when you stop training or take a break. Make sure you train regularly enough so that you don't start losing condition or plateauing.

### FACTOR IN DAILY LIFE

Consider how much time you can commit to per week without it having a negative effect on your work, family life, or friendships. Also decide when you'll do your training: are you an early riser who trains best in the morning, or a night owl who prefers to train in the evening? Do your training times impact on others? To avoid causing yourself unnecessary problems and meeting with resistance from those closest to you, ensure that your programme fits in as harmoniously as possible with your normal daily life.

### KEEP A TRAINING LOG

It's easy to forget the details of a day's training. But if you keep a training log, you can flick through it to remind yourself which sessions were especially tough or enjoyable. A log can be a terrific motivator, allowing you to see how hard you've worked, how consistent you've been, and how you've progressed. You can keep detailed records if you like, but you can boost your spirits even by just recording the session, how you felt before, during, and after, and your times. (See also pp.132-133.)

# YOUR PROFILE

**The better you understand** your own abilities, the better you can tailor your training. Performance profiling is all about assessing your strengths and weaknesses, and knowing where, by triathlon standards, you currently stand. Your profile, whether simple or complex, should give you a clear idea of the areas in which you're weakest. You can then use your profile to create a training plan that will develop your abilities in those weaker areas.

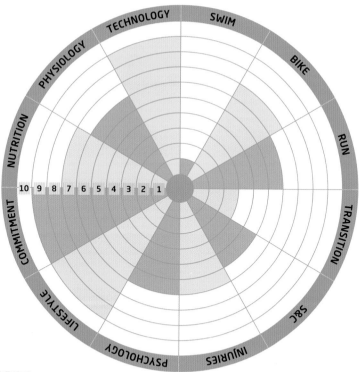

## YOUR STRENGTHS AND WEAKNESSES

If you regularly test your performance (see pp.28-29, 50-51, 78-79), you'll have good statistics to compare against fitness charts to see how you're doing. You can add as many segments as you like to your profile, but the 12 shown here will give you a good overall picture of your abilities. Don't worry if, when you start, you're scoring at the lower end of the scale in most segments - after all, improvement is what training's for. Plotting your scores now will mean that in six months' time you will feel hugely encouraged when you see your progress.

**This performance profile** shows typical scores for someone new to triathlon who is sporty, likes cycling and running, but has done little or no swimming. The list below gives an idea of how each segment is assessed, with a typical novice's scores in bold type.

**KEY:**

1 = POOR
10 = BEST IN YOUR AGE GROUP/CLASS

**SWIM** Elite athletes compare themselves with the best in the world, but how do you compare with your age group? **(Sample score: 1/10)**

**BIKE** How do you compare with your age group? **(7/10)**

**RUN** How do you compare with your age group? **(6/10)**

**TRANSITION** Can you transition from swim to bike and from bike to run quickly and smoothly compared with your peers? **(3/10)**

**STRENGTH AND CONDITIONING (S&C)** How does each part of your body perform during training and racing? **(5/10)**

**INJURY RATE/ROBUSTNESS** How often do you get injured? **(6/10)**

**PSYCHOLOGY** How do you deal with "no man's land"? **(6/10)**

**LIFESTYLE** Do you sleep well? Are you happy? Are you stressed? **(9/10)**

**COMMITMENT** How is your day-to-day commitment to your training? **(9/10)**

**NUTRITION** Do you have a healthy diet and a good understanding of nutrition and hydration? **(7/10)**

**PHYSIOLOGY** How is your VO2 max, for example? If you do one of the tests on p.79 and check the charts on pp.158-159, how does your score compare with others in your age group? **(6/10)**

**TECHNOLOGY** Do you measure power and cadence, and upload data for analysis? Do you understand your bike's set-up and gearing? How good is your bike maintenance? **(9/10)**

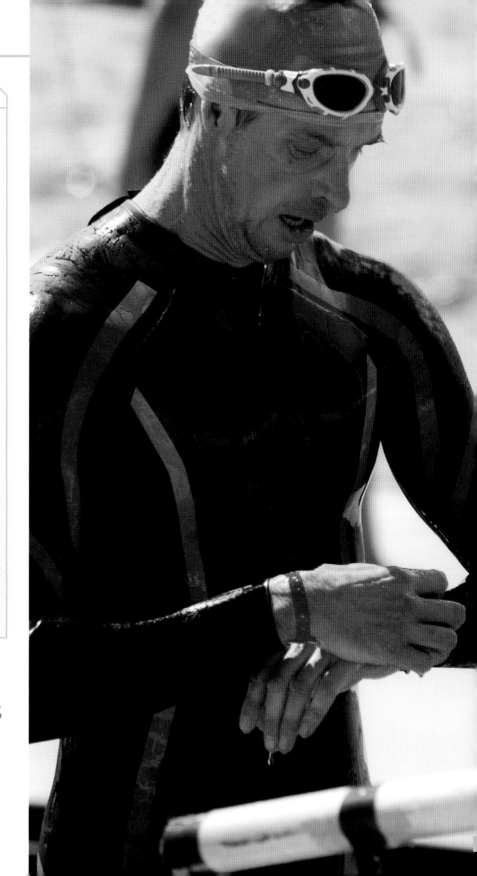

## DRILLING DOWN

Once you've made your profile and established your current levels, you can then break down each discipline into individual skills and abilities.

### SWIM
- Stroke cycle / technique
- Sprint
- Rounding buoys
- Staying on feet / drafting
- Sighting
- Pace judgement
- Endurance
- Robustness / injury rate
- Getting out of trouble
- Exiting water
- Running to bike

### BIKE
- Technique and cadence
- Time trialling
- Cornering
- Endurance
- Hill climbing
- Pace judgement
- Concentration
- Robustness / injury rate
- Bike set-up
- Maintenance

### RUN
- Technique and strike rate
- Endurance
- Hill running
- Pace judgement
- Dealing with "no man's land"
- Concentration
- Sprint finish
- Robustness / injury rate

**❝ WHAT YOU CHOOSE** TO INCLUDE IN **YOUR PROFILE** IS UP TO YOU. EVERYONE HAS THEIR **WEAK POINTS**; IF YOU KEEP AN EYE ON YOURS, YOU CAN WORK ON THEM UNTIL THEY **NO LONGER HINDER** YOUR PROGRESS. ❞

# PLANNING YOUR TRAINING

**Whether you're an elite pro** or a complete novice, you should adopt the same approach to planning your triathlon training: start with an end goal in mind and work back from there to devise a structured schedule. You may have your eye on one major Ironman or several races over the summer, but whatever your goal, think ahead.

**6**

THE AVERAGE NUMBER OF WEEKS IT TAKES TO ADOPT A NEW TECHNIQUE OR MOVEMENT

## YOUR ROUTE TO SUCCESS

### SELECT YOUR "A" RACE

In triathlon, the race that you are specifically building up to is called the "A" race. Plan your peak and tapering (see pp.138-139) around its date to ensure your performance is at its very best on the day. Your B races are similar to the A race, but you only do a short taper for them, while for a C race you just keep training through it. Decide at the outset what your A race will be, then build your training programme backwards from there.

### INCORPORATE SOME R&R

When we train, we force our bodies to adapt to new physical demands. These adaptations actually occur while we're recovering, so schedule in at least one rest day a week and a recovery week every fourth week. You won't stop training altogether in a recovery week, but you should reduce your efforts to 50-60 per cent of the previous week's training and take about three rest days.

### FOUNDATION PHASE

Don't worry about improving your speed and times in this phase – focus on mastering any technical issues you may have. Since the race isn't looming just yet, you can relax and work on the mechanics of your swimming, running, and cycling, addressing issues that are holding you back and getting yourself into better habits. You are also teaching your body to become fat-adapted (using fat as fuel) in your training sessions as the level of intensity increases – gradually building up over 8-12 weeks from Level 1 (Easy) to Level 2 and Level 3 (see pp.160-161). Then you'll be ready to hit the winter phase of training with energy and enthusiasm. For a sample foundation programme, see pp.122-123.

# TIMING YOUR ABC

Your A race schedule takes priority when planning your season. Always factor in time, effort, goals, and abilities when selecting this race. No matter what level of athlete you are, to get the best out of yourself you will need to go through three basic phases of training – foundation, winter, and race-season preparation – and each is 8-12 weeks long. For sample training programmes for Sprint, Olympic, Half Ironman, and Ironman, see pp.124-131.

| TYPE OF RACE | PURPOSE |
| --- | --- |
| A | Your main race of the season; the one you specifically train for so that you can deliver on race day. All your training sessions are geared towards optimum performance at this race. |
| B | This is a supporting race to test your fitness. It involves less tapering and takes place during the build-up to your main event, or possibly after. |
| C | This should be convenient and fun, requiring effort but without the worry about finishing times. Treat it as a brick session (one that combines all three sports), either early or late in the season. |

## WINTER PHASE

During this second phase, look to work hard on all elements of your fitness, especially if you're working up to a 70.3 or Ironman. In most countries, this phase is done in winter. In the severe winters of the northern hemisphere, it takes grit to get out there and train. But think of it this way: every time you train in nasty conditions, you're putting pennies in your psychological bank that you can draw on if race day is tough.

As you progressively increase the volume of your training, remember to follow the 10 per cent principle (see p.116). You need to go into the preparation phase not exhausted but excited to get out and do the specific training required for your big race of the year.

## PREPARATION PHASE

At around 12 weeks before your A race, revisit your performance profile to assess your strengths and weaknesses (see pp.118-119). Now prioritize what you need to do in your training and tapering to bring your body and mind to peak fitness prior to your A race. This is where specificity (see p.116) truly kicks in:

- Sprint distance: prioritize strength, VO2 (see pp.78-79), and some max pace work
- Olympic: prioritize strength, endurance, and VO2
- Half Ironman (70.3): prioritize endurance, force work, and a little VO2
- Ironman: prioritize endurance and force work on the bike

Be realistic. If you've been ill or had an injury, build slowly and sensibly back up to full training. A week off training won't affect your overall conditioning, so don't then rush back and make yourself ill again. Adapt your training accordingly.

## MAINTENANCE PHASE

Leading up to your A race, you will be training hard, eating well, and foregoing some treats. Once the race is over you can reward yourself, but remember to stay active. If you keep your body ticking over with walking or light swimming, you'll feel the benefit when it's time to train hard again. Many elite athletes follow this simple formula:

- Day one: swim
- Day two: swim and bike
- Day three: swim, bike, and run

Keep it light and stress-free, especially after Olympic-distance racing. If you have done an Ironman, listen to your body in the post-race euphoria – it may take a while for the full impact to make itself felt. Then reassess your performance profile, work on your technique, and plan for another race – or ease off until the end of the season and start looking forward to next year!

# FOUNDATION PROGRAMME

**Before you begin your training** for your chosen distance (Sprint, Olympic, 70.3, or Ironman), you first need to complete an 8-12 week foundation phase. The sample programme opposite is designed to build your technique, strength, and fitness, and will help you avoid injury in the run-up to race day.

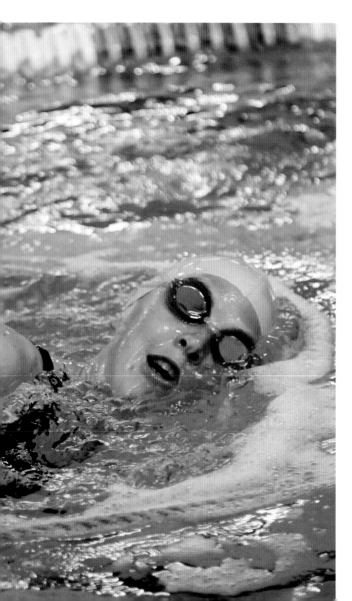

## KEY »

For more details on the training sessions and levels shown in the sample foundation programme opposite, see the following pages:

| | |
|---|---|
| **Swim** training | pp.20-27 |
| **Bike** training | pp.46-49 |
| **Run** training | pp.68-77 |
| **Strength and conditioning (S&C)** | pp.94-102 |
| **Levels (L)** | pp.160-161 |
| **Drills** | see training, above |

## KEY ELEMENTS OF THE PROGRAMME

The triathlon year is a long one and in order to avoid over- exhaustion in the first few months, you should build up progressively. As the foundation phase takes place outside the racing season, your training sessions should be more relaxed, with the focus on mastering the mechanics of swimming, cycling, and running, drills for key skills, warm-up techniques, and strength and conditioning exercises.

1 **ECONOMY OF MOTION** You are training your body to move efficiently to the best of your ability, with minimum oxygen consumption for a given speed.

2 **PRACTICE** When making significant changes to your technique, stay focused and repeat the movement patterns as often as you can. It will take at least three sessions a week over six weeks to see the required changes.

3 **PROGRESSION** The foundation programme is structured to increase the level of difficulty gradually, through volume, intensity, or frequency of training. Try to build up your training gradually from the first four weeks shown opposite; don't increase it by more than 10 per cent a week.

4 **PERFORMANCE PROFILING** It's important to tailor any training plan to your particular level and ability; knowing exactly how far to push yourself will reduce the risk of illness and injury. The foundation programme will help you assess your current level of fitness and gradually build on it.

5 **FAT ADAPTATION** Your body will start to learn how to utliize its fat more effectively through a combination of training and nutrition (see pp.90-91). Training your body to use fat as a source of energy early on will help to improve your performance later, as the programme intensifies.

| WEEK/TIME | | MONDAY | TUESDAY | WEDNESDAY | THURSDAY | FRIDAY | SATURDAY | SUNDAY | TOTAL TIME |
|---|---|---|---|---|---|---|---|---|---|
| 1 | AM: | **Swim** L1/2, 30 mins, **Drills** | **Bike** L2, 45 mins, **Drills** | **Swim** L2, 40 mins | **Bike** L2, 40 mins | Rest day | **Swim** L1/2, 40 mins | **Bike** L1/2, 90 mins | c.8 hrs |
| | PM: | **Run** L2, 20 mins warm-up and 10 x 30 secs | **S&C** Phase 1 30 mins | **Run** L2, 45 mins | **S&C** Phase 1 30 mins | | **Run** L1/2, 40 mins | | |
| 2 | AM: | **Swim** L1/2, 30 mins, **Drills** | **Bike** L2, 45 mins, **Drills** | **Swim** L2, 40 mins | **Bike** L2, 40 mins | Rest day | **Swim** L1/2, 45 mins | **Bike** L1/2, 105 mins | c.8.5 hrs |
| | PM: | **Run** L2, 20 mins warm-up and 15 x 30 secs | **S&C** Phase 1 30 mins | **Run** L3, 45 mins | **S&C** Phase 1 30 mins | | **Run** L1/2, 40 mins | | |
| 3 | AM: | **Swim** L1/2, 30 mins, **Drills** | **Bike** L2, 45 mins, **Drills** | **Swim** L2, 40 mins | **Bike** L2, 40 mins | Rest day | **Swim** L1/2, 60 mins | **Bike** L1, 2 hrs | c.9 hrs |
| | PM: | **Run** L2, 20 mins warm-up and 10 x 45 secs | **S&C** Phase 1 30 mins | **Run** L3, 45 mins | **S&C** Phase 1 30 mins | | **Run** L1/2, 50 mins | | |
| 4 | AM: | Rest day | **Bike** L2, 30 mins into 20 mins **run** off bike | **Swim** L2, 40 mins | **Bike** L3, 40 mins | Rest day | **Swim** L1/2, 40 mins | Rest day | c.5 hrs |
| | PM: | | **S&C** Phase 1 30 mins | **Run** L3, 45 mins | **S&C** Phase 1 30 mins | | **Run** L1/2, 40 mins | | |

Repeat Weeks 1–4 two to three times in total, increasing your volume of training overall by no more than 10 per cent per week.

# SPRINT PROGRAMME

**Swim 750m - Bike 20km - Run 5km** If you are new to triathlon, the sprint distance is the shortest and perhaps the easiest to start with. While you can push your body really hard during the sprint, working at high levels of intensity, the end of each leg is not too far off. If this is your first triathlon and you just want to get round, don't overdo it in your preparation phase: adapt this sample 12-week programme to your needs.

## KEY »

For details on the training sessions and levels shown in the programme opposite, see the following pages:

| | | |
|---|---|---|
| S | **Swim** training | pp.20-27 |
| B | **Bike** training | pp.46-49 |
| R | **Run** training | pp.68-77 |
| S&C | **Strength and Conditioning Phase 3** | pp.112-113 |
| L | **Level** | pp.160-161 |
| D | **Drills** | see training, above |

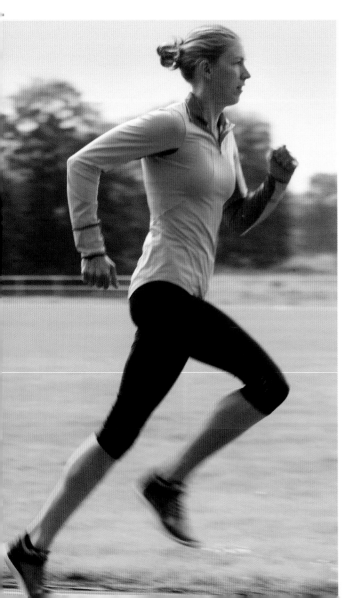

## TRAINING INTENSITY

The sprint programme includes several high-intensity sessions at Levels 4 and 5. If you are fit, you can push your body harder for short periods of time during the sprint, but this involves a little more lactate production and pain: the high-intensity sessions will help prepare your body to perform close to your lactate threshold level (see pp.160-161). However, if you just want to complete the race, you don't need high-intensity training sessions to do that. Remember this is a sample programme – tailor your training to fit your needs.

## THE PROGRAMME

In order to reduce the risk of injury, you must first complete the foundation phase of training (see pp.122-123). This will help eliminate any technical weaknesses so that you fully benefit from your preparation phase. If you already have a good basic level of fitness, then you can focus on building towards the higher-intensity sessions, but make sure that you progress at a gradual rate, and follow the 10 per cent rule (see p.116).

## YOUR GOALS

Elite athletes typically complete sprint distances in under an hour. Mid-pack athletes will probably take about 80 minutes or longer to finish. If this is your first triathlon, your main aim could be to get around the course and complete it successfully. Remember you are really only competing against yourself. The most important thing about the race is to have fun.

| WEEK/TIME | | MONDAY | TUESDAY | WEDNESDAY | THURSDAY | FRIDAY | SATURDAY | SUNDAY | TOTAL TIME |
|---|---|---|---|---|---|---|---|---|---|
| 1 | AM: | S L4, 60 mins | B L2, 45 mins, D | S L5, 60 mins | B L3, 60 mins | Rest day | S L3, 40 mins | B L1/2, 90 mins | c.9.5 hrs |
| | PM: | R L5, 40 mins | S&C 30 mins | R L4, 60 mins | S&C 30 mins | | R L1/2, 60 mins | | |
| 2 | AM: | S L5, 60 mins | B L2, 45 mins, D | S L4, 60 mins | B L3, 60 mins | Rest day | S L1/2, 40 mins | B L3, 100 mins into 10 mins R off B L1 | c.9.5 hrs |
| | PM: | R L4, 45 mins | S&C 30 mins | R L5, 60 mins | S&C 30 mins | | R L1/2, 40 mins | | |
| 3 | AM: | S L1/2, 60 mins, D | B L2, 45 mins, D | S L4, 60 mins | B L4, 60 mins | Rest day | S L3, 40 mins | B L2, 100 mins into 15 mins R off B L1 | c.10 hrs |
| | PM: | R L5, 45 mins | S&C 30 mins | R L3, 60 mins | S&C 30 mins | | R L1/2, 50 mins | | |
| 4 Recovery week | AM: | Rest day | B L4, 30 mins into 20 mins R off B L2 | S L2, 40 mins | B L3, 40 mins | Rest day | S L5, 40 mins | Rest day | c.5 hrs |
| | PM: | | S&C 30 mins | R L3, 45 mins | S&C 30 mins | | R L5, hills, 40 mins | | |
| 5 | AM: | S L4, 60 mins | B L2, 45 mins, D | S L5, 60 mins | B L3, 60 mins | Rest day | S L2/3, 40 mins | B L2, 100 mins into 15 mins R off B L1 | c.10 hrs |
| | PM: | R L5, 45 mins | S&C 30 mins | R L3, 60 mins | S&C 30 mins | | R L2, 50 mins | | |
| 6 | AM: | S L2, 60 mins, D | B L2, 45 mins, D | S L4, 60 mins | B L4, 60 mins | Rest day | S L1/2, 40 mins | B L2, 110 mins into 20 mins R off B L1 | c.10.5 hrs |
| | PM: | R L5, 45 mins | S&C 30 mins | R L3, 60 mins | S&C 30 mins | | R L2, 60 mins | | |
| 7 | AM: | S L5, 60 mins | B L2, 45 mins, D | S L4, 60 mins | B L3, 60 mins | Rest day | S L3, 40 mins | B L2, 110 mins into 10 mins R off B L1 | c.10.5 hrs |
| | PM: | R L5, 45 mins | S&C 30 mins | R L3, 60 mins | S&C 30 mins | | R L2, 70 mins | | |
| 8 Recovery week | AM: | Rest day | B L4, 30 mins into 20 mins R off B L1 | S L2, 40 mins | B L3, 40 mins | Rest day | S L5, 40 mins | Rest day | c.5 hrs |
| | PM: | | S&C 30 mins | R L3, 45 mins | S&C 30 mins | | R L4, hills, 40 mins | | |
| 9 | AM: | S L5, 60 mins | B L2, 45 mins, D | S L4, 60 mins | B L4, 60 mins | Rest day | S L2, 60 mins | B L2, 120 mins | c.10.5 hrs |
| | PM: | R L4, 45 mins | S&C 30 mins | R L5, 60 mins | S&C 30 mins | | R L1, 70 mins | | |
| 10 | AM: | S L2-5, 60 mins | B L2, 45 mins, D | S L2/3, 60 mins | B L3/4, 60 mins | Rest day | S L1, 60 mins | B L1, 90 mins, 20 mins R off B build from L2 to 5k pace L3 | c.9 hrs |
| | PM: | R L4, 30 mins | S&C 30 mins | R L3, 45 mins | S&C 30 mins | | Rest | | |
| 11 | AM: | S L2-5, 60 mins | B L2, 45 mins, D | S L2/3, 45 mins | B L3/4, 40mins | START TAPER ← | S L1, 60 mins | B L1, 60 mins, 20 mins R off B build from L1 to 5k pace | c.7 hrs |
| | PM: | R L4, 30 mins | S&C 15 mins trunk only | R L3 race pace work, 45 mins | S&C 10 mins trunk only | Rest day | Rest | | |
| 12 Race Week | AM: | Rest day if feeling tired; if not, S | B L2, 30 mins into 20 mins R off B | S L2, 40 mins | B L3, 40 mins | Rest day or light S 20 mins | S pick ups L1-3, 20 mins B pick ups L1-3, 30 mins R pick ups L1-3, 20 mins | **RACE DAY** S 750m B 20km R 5km | c.6 hrs |
| | PM: | 40 mins | S&C 10 mins, trunk only | R L3, 45 mins | Rest | | | | |

# OLYMPIC PROGRAMME

**Swim 1500m - Bike 40km - Run 10km** Many athletes find the Olympic triathlon the hardest distance: pushing the body's aerobic threshold, it demands physical and mental toughness. The sample Olympic programme opposite builds on the foundation phase to help you rise to the challenge.

## KEY »

For details on the training sessions and levels shown in the programme opposite, see the following pages:

| | | |
|---|---|---|
| S | **Swim** training | pp.20-27 |
| B | **Bike** training | pp.46-49 |
| R | **Run** training | pp.68-77 |
| S&C | **Strength and Conditioning Phase 3** | pp.112-113 |
| L | **Level** | pp.160-161 |
| D | **Drills** | see training, above |

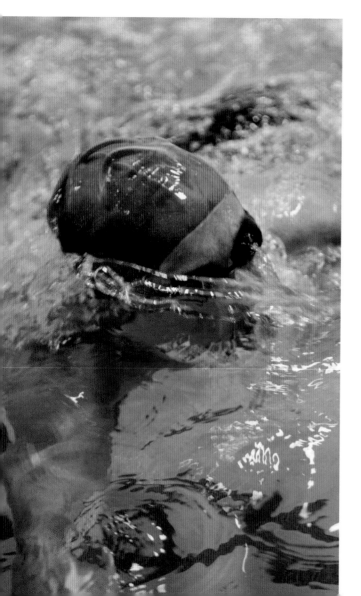

## TRAINING INTENSITY

The Olympic programme is designed to build your strength endurance. The work schedule is similar to the sprint programme, with sessions across different levels of intensity, but you will be asked to swim, bike, and run for longer, in order to build both physical and mental strength.

## BUILDING ON A FIRM FOUNDATION

As with the sprint programme, a basic level of fitness is essential for the Olympic programme. If this is your first Olympic triathlon, then it is crucial that you follow the foundation course first (see pp.122-123). The foundation phase allows you to work on the mechanics of your swimming, running, and cycling, and ensures you progress safely throughout the training programme, minimizing the risk of injury. Remember, too, that the sample programme opposite is a guideline and adapt it to your individual needs.

## YOUR GOALS

Elite male athletes will complete an Olympic triathlon in under two hours; female athletes will not be far behind. A mid-pack athlete will typically complete this distance in about two and a half hours. This race is about mental fortitude as well as endurance, so pacing is key: the distances are demanding and the speed of each stage is fast, so you'll need to strike a balance between lasting the distance and racing it hard. First-timers should just get a feel for the pace, trust their training, and focus on a strong race.

| WEEK/TIME | | MONDAY | TUESDAY | WEDNESDAY | THURSDAY | FRIDAY | SATURDAY | SUNDAY | TOTAL TIME |
|---|---|---|---|---|---|---|---|---|---|
| 1 | AM: | S L3, 60 mins | B L2, 45 mins, D | S L4, 60 mins | B L4, 60 mins | Rest day | S L1/2, 60 mins | B L1/2, 120 mins | c.10.5 hrs |
| | PM: | R L5, 40 mins | S&C 30 mins | R L4, 60 mins | S&C 30 mins | | R L1/2, 60 mins | | |
| 2 | AM: | S L2, 60 mins, D | B L2, 60 mins, D | S L4, 60 mins | B L4, 60 mins | Rest day | S L1/2, 60 mins | B L1/2, 120 mins into 10 mins R off B L1 | c.10.5 hrs |
| | PM: | R L4, 40 mins | S&C 30 mins | R L3, 60 mins | S&C 30 mins | | R L3, 40 mins | | |
| 3 | AM: | S L3, 60 mins, D | B L2, 60 mins, D | S L4, 60 mins | B L4, 60 mins | Rest day | S L1/2, 70 mins | B L3, 90mins into 15 mins R off B L1 | c.11 hrs |
| | PM: | R L4, 50 mins | S&C 30 mins | R L4, 60 mins | S&C 30 mins | | R L1/2, 70 mins | | |
| 4 Recovery week | AM: | Rest day | B L4, 30 mins into 20 mins R off B L1 | S L2, 40 mins | B L3, 40 mins | Rest day | S L5, 60 mins | Rest day | c.5 hrs |
| | PM: | | S&C 30 mins | R L3, 45 mins | S&C 30 mins | | R or B L4 60 mins | | |
| 5 | AM: | S L5, 60 mins, D | B L2, 50 mins, D | S L4, 60 mins | B L3, 60 mins | Rest day | S L1/2, 60 mins | B L1/2, 140 mins | c.11 hrs |
| | PM: | R L5, 50 mins | S&C 30 mins | R L4, 60 mins | S&C 30 mins | | R L3, 60 mins | | |
| 6 | AM: | S L2, 60 mins, D | B L2, 60 mins, D | S L5, 60 mins | B L3, 60 mins | Rest day | S L1/2, 60 mins | B L3, 90 mins, into 10 mins R off B L1 | c.11 hrs |
| | PM: | R L3, 60 mins | S&C 30 mins | R L4, 60 mins | S&C 30 mins | | R L1/2, 80 mins | | |
| 7 | AM: | S L4, 60 mins | B L2, 45 mins, D | S L5, 60 mins | B L3, 60 mins | Rest day | S L1/2, 60 mins | B L1/2, 160 mins | c.11 hrs |
| | PM: | R L5, 45 mins | S&C 30 mins | R L4, 60 mins | S&C 30 mins | | R L3, 50 mins | | |
| 8 Recovery week | AM: | Rest day | B L4, 30 mins into 20 mins R off B L1 | S L2, 60 mins | B L3, 40 mins | Rest day | S L4, 60 mins | Rest day | c.6.5 hrs |
| | PM: | | S&C 30 mins | R L3, 45 mins | S&C 30 mins | | R or B L3 75 mins | | |
| 9 | AM: | S L5, 60 mins, D | B L2, 45 mins, D | S L3, 60 mins | B L3, 60 mins | Rest day | S L1/2, 30 mins | B L2/3, 180 mins | c.11.5 hrs |
| | PM: | R L5, 45 mins | S&C 30 mins | R L4, 60 mins | S&C 30 mins | | R L1/2, 90 mins | | |
| 10 | AM: | S L2, 60 mins, D | B L2, 60 mins, D | S L5, 60 mins | B L3/4, 60 mins | Rest day | S L3, 60 mins | B L1, 90mins, 30 mins R off B build from L2 to 10k pace L3 | c.9 hrs |
| | PM: | Rest | S&C 30 mins | R L3, 60 mins race pace work | S&C 30 mins | | Rest | | |
| 11 | AM: | S L5, 60 mins | B L2, 45 mins D | S L2/3, 60 mins | B L3/4, 40 mins | START TAPER ← | S L1, 60 mins | B L1, 60 mins, 20 mins R off B build from L1 to 5k pace | c.8 hrs |
| | PM: | R L4, 60 mins | S&C 15 mins, trunk only | R L3, 60 mins race pace work | S&C 10 mins, trunk only | Rest day | Rest | | |
| 12 Recovery week | AM: | S, 40 mins recovery, D | B L2, 30 mins into 20 mins R off B L1 | S L3, 40 mins | B L3, 40 mins | Rest day or light S 20 mins | S pick-ups L1-3, 20 mins B pick-ups L1-3, 30 mins R pick-ups L1-3, 15 mins | RACE DAY S 1500m B 40km R 10km | c.7 hrs |
| | PM: | | S&C 10 mins, trunk only | R L3, 45 mins | Rest | | | | |

# HALF IRONMAN PROGRAMME (70.3)

**Swim 1900m - Bike 90km - Run 21km** The Half Ironman (also known as 70.3) is a test of endurance and aerobic capacity. Planning your fuelling strategy for this distance is the key to success: you need enough energy to meet the demands of each leg or you run the risk of "running on empty" at the end.

**KEY »**

For details on the training sessions and levels shown in the programme opposite, see the following pages:

| | | |
|---|---|---|
| S | **Swim** training | pp.20-27 |
| B | **Bike** training | pp.46-49 |
| R | **Run** training | pp.68-77 |
| S&C | **Strength and Conditioning Phase 3** | pp.112-113 |
| L | **Level** | pp.160-161 |
| D | **Drills** | see training, above |

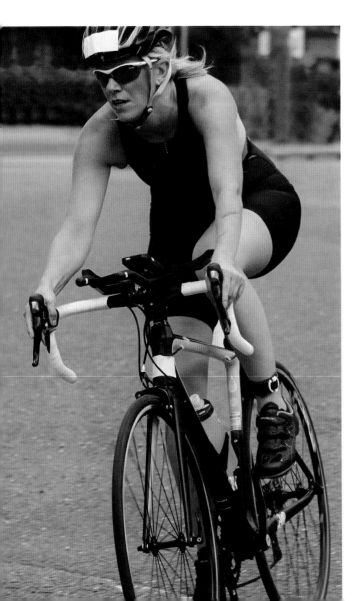

## TRAINING INTENSITY

The Half Ironman is a greater test of endurance than Sprint and Olympic triathlons, so the sample 12-week training programme opposite places more emphasis on distance in the run and bike sessions, and less on high intensity. Working more at Level 3 will help to increase your aerobic capacity (see pp.160-161) and train your body to use energy more efficiently. A key outcome of your training is the ability to endure a bike intensity close to your aerobic threshold while mentally dealing with the half marathon still to come.

## NO HALF MEASURES

The Half Ironman programme is taxing on the body, so you must complete the foundation phase (see pp.122-123) before embarking on the rest of your training. Only increase the duration of a session or your total volume each week by about 10 per cent from your previous session or week. The Half Ironman programme includes one rest day a week to allow your body time to recover, three rest days in a recovery week, and tapering at the end to prepare your body for race day (see pp.138-139).

## YOUR GOALS

Elite male athletes complete this distance in about 4 hours 15 minutes; females in about 4 hours 30 minutes. Mid-pack athletes typically finish in about 5 hours 30 minutes. Adequate nutrition and hydration are essential for the Half Ironman, so make sure you have worked out optimum fuelling strategy for this distance on race day (see pp.142-143).

| WEEK/TIME | | MONDAY | TUESDAY | WEDNESDAY | THURSDAY | FRIDAY | SATURDAY | SUNDAY | TOTAL TIME |
|---|---|---|---|---|---|---|---|---|---|
| 1 | AM: | S L3, 60 mins, D | B L2, 45 mins, D | S L4, 60 mins | B L4, 60 mins | Rest day | S L1/2, 60 mins | B L1, 120 mins | c.11 hrs |
| | PM: | R L3, 60 mins | S&C 30 mins | R L4, 60 mins | S&C 30 mins | | R L1/2, 80 mins | | |
| 2 | AM: | S L3, 60 mins, D | B L2, 45 mins, D | S L4, 60 mins | B L4, 60 mins | Rest day | S L1/2, 75 mins | B L2, 180 mins | c.12 hrs |
| | PM: | R L4, 40 mins | S&C 30 mins | R L4, 60 mins | S&C 30 mins | | R L/2, 60 mins | | |
| 3 | AM: | S L3, 60 mins, D | B L2, 45 mins, D | S L4, 60 mins | B L4, 60 mins | Rest day | S L1/2, 90 mins | B L2, 150 mins | c.12 hrs |
| | PM: | R L4, 45 mins | S&C 30 mins | R L4, 60 mins | S&C 30 mins | | R L1/2, 90 mins | | |
| 4 Recovery week | AM: | Rest day | B L4, 60 mins into 20 mins R off B L1 | S L2, 60 mins | B L3, 60 mins | Rest day | S L1/2, 90 mins | Rest day | c.6.5 hrs |
| | PM: | | S&C 15 mins | R L3, 65 mins | S&C 15 mins | | R or B L4, 60 mins | | |
| 5 | AM: | S L3, 60 mins, D | B L2, 40 mins, D | S L4, 60 mins | B L4, 60 mins | Rest day | S L1/2, 60 mins | B L2, 210 mins | c.12 hrs |
| | PM: | R L4, 60 mins | S&C 30 mins | R L4, 60 mins | S&C 15 mins | | R L1/2, 60 mins | | |
| 6 | AM: | S L2, 60 mins, D | B L2, 60 mins, D | S L2, 60 mins | B L3, 60 mins | Rest day | S L1/2, 75 mins | B L3, 130 mins | c.12 hrs |
| | PM: | R L4, 60 mins | S&C 30 mins | R L3, 60 mins | S&C 30 mins | | R L1/2, 105 mins | | |
| 7 | AM: | S L2, 60 mins, D | B L2, 40 mins, D | S L4, 60 mins | B L3, 60 mins | Rest day | S L2, 45 mins | B L2, 240 mins | c.12 hrs |
| | PM: | R L3, 60 mins | S&C 30 mins | R L3/4, 60 mins | S&C 15 mins | | R L2, 60 mins | | |
| 8 Recovery week | AM: | Rest day | B L4, 60 mins into 20 mins R off B L1 | S L2, 60 mins | B L3, 60 mins | Rest day | S L1/2, 90 mins | Rest day | c.6.5 hrs |
| | PM: | | S&C 15 mins | R L3, 65 mins | S&C 15 mins | | R or B L4, 60 mins | | |
| 9 | AM: | S L2, 60 mins, D | B L2, 60 mins, D | S L2, 60 mins | B L3, 60 mins | Rest day | S L1/2, 75 mins | B L2, 120 mins | c.12 hrs |
| | PM: | R L4, 45 mins | S&C 30 mins | R L3, 75 mins | S&C 30 mins | | R L1/2, 120 mins | | |
| 10 | AM: | S L2, 60 mins | B L2, 45 mins, D | S L5, 60 mins | B L3/4, 60 mins | Rest day | S L3, 90 mins | B L1, 210 mins into 15 mins R off B | c.11.5 hrs |
| | PM: | R L1/2, 30 mins | S&C 30 mins | R L2, 90 mins | S&C 15 mins | | Rest | | |
| 11 | AM: | S L4, 60 mins | B L2, 45 mins, D | S L3, 45 mins | B L3, 60 mins | START TAPER ← | S L2, 75 mins | B 90 mins, into 20 mins R off B start L1, build to 5k pace | c.9 hrs |
| | PM: | R L4, 45 mins | S&C 15 mins, trunk only | R L2/3, 75 mins race pace work | S&C 10 mins, trunk only | Rest day | Rest | | |
| 12 Race week | AM: | S 40 mins | B L2, 60 mins into 20 mins R off B L1 | S L3, 40 mins | B L3, 40 mins into R 10 mins | Rest day | S pick-ups L1-3, 20 mins B pick-ups L1-3, 30 mins R pick-ups L1-3, 20 mins | RACE DAY S 1900m B 90km R 21km | c.8 hrs |
| | PM: | | S&C 10 mins | | Rest | | | | |

# IRONMAN PROGRAMME

**Swim 3.8km - Bike 180km - Run 42km** Ironman is the greatest endurance test of all, and your training requires total focus and self-discipline. Prepare properly, build steadily, and reap the glory when you cross that finishing line.

**KEY »**

For details on the training sessions and levels shown in the programme opposite, see the following pages:

| | | |
|---|---|---|
| S | **Swim** training | pp.20-27 |
| B | **Bike** training | pp.46-49 |
| R | **Run** training | pp.68-77 |
| S&C | **Strength and Conditioning Phase 3** | pp.112-113 |
| L | **Level** | pp.160-161 |
| D | **Drills** | see training |

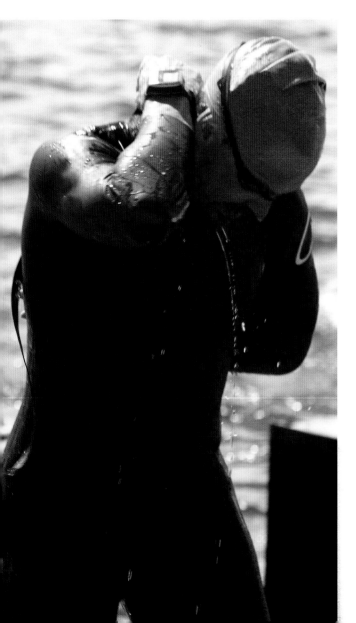

## TRAINING INTENSITY

Ironman is a long way. In the sample programme opposite, the duration of the sessions across all three disciplines increases progressively over a minimum 12 weeks. There is a considerable amount of work in the Level 1 and Level 2 zones, and you will need to build steadily to avoid injury. Precision fuelling is also very important, so use your training to experiment with optimum nutrition and hydration (see pp.88–91).

## FIRST STEPS

Any athlete who takes on this distance must be robust, so fitness is crucial before embarking on the Ironman programme. First complete the foundation phase (see pp.122-123), then focus your winter phase primarily on improving your fitness rather than doing exhausting mega mileage. You need to go into your preparation phase feeling excited about the specific work required for your big race of the year.

## YOUR GOALS

Ironman is the most challenging distance of all and finishing the course is a huge achievement. The race day lasts about 10-14 hours (longer than the sprint, Olympic, and Half Ironman combined). Elite male athletes typically complete this race in about 8 hours and 30 minutes; females in about 9 hours and 15 minutes. Mid-pack athletes take between 10 hours 45 minutes and 12 hours, with the cut-off being 17 hours. It takes many months of dedicated training to prepare for an Ironman, so stay focused. When you finish the race, the spectators will shout "You are an Ironman!"

| WEEK/TIME | | MONDAY | TUESDAY | WEDNESDAY | THURSDAY | FRIDAY | SATURDAY | SUNDAY | TOTAL TIME |
|---|---|---|---|---|---|---|---|---|---|
| 1 | AM: | S L3, 60 mins, **D** | B L2, 45 mins, **D** | S L4, 60 mins | B L3, 60 mins | Rest day | S L1/2, 60 mins | B L3, 120 mins | c.11.5 hrs |
| | PM: | R L3, 45 mins | S&C 30 mins | R L3, 60 mins | S&C 30 mins | | R L1/2, 80 mins | | |
| 2 | AM: | S L3, 60 mins, **D** | B L2, 50 mins, **D** | S L4, 60 mins | B L4, 60 mins | Rest day | S L1/2, 75 mins | B L1/2, 180 mins | c.12 hrs |
| | PM: | R L2, 40 mins | S&C 30 mins | R L3, 60 mins | S&C 30 mins | | R L3, 60 mins | | |
| 3 | AM: | S L3, 60mins, **D** | B L2, 60 mins, **D** | S L4, 60 mins | B L3, 60 mins | Rest day | S L1/2, 90 mins | B L3, 150 mins | c.12 hrs |
| | PM: | R L2, 60 mins | S&C 30 mins | R L3, 90 mins | S&C 30 mins | | R L1/2, 90 mins | | |
| 4 Recovery week | AM: | Rest day | B L4, 60mins into 20 mins R off **B** L1 | S L2, 60 mins | B L3, 60 mins | Rest day | S L1/2, 90 mins | Rest day | c.6.5 hrs |
| | PM: | | S&C 30mins | R L3, 65mins | S&C 30mins | | R L4, 60mins | | |
| 5 | AM: | S L3, 60 mins **D** | B L2, 40 mins **D** | S L4, 60 mins | B L3, 60 mins | Rest day | S L1/2, 90 mins | B L1/2, 210 mins | c.12.5 hrs |
| | PM: | R L2, 60 mins | S&C 30 mins | R L3, 60 mins | S&C 30 mins | | R L3, 60 mins | | |
| 6 | AM: | S L2, 60 mins, **D** | B L2, 60 mins, **D** | S L2, 60 mins | B L3, 60 mins | Rest day | S L1/2, 90 mins | B L3, 150 mins | c.13 hrs |
| | PM: | R L2, 60 mins | S&C 30 mins | R L3, 60 mins | S&C 30 mins | | R L1/2, 105 mins | | |
| 7 | AM: | S L2, 60 mins, **D** | B L2, 40 mins, **D** | S L4, 60 mins | B L3, 60 mins | Rest day | S L2, 90 mins | B L1/2, 240 mins | c.13 hrs |
| | PM: | R L2, 60 mins | S&C 30 mins | R L3, 60 mins | S&C 30 mins | | R L3, 60 mins | | |
| 8 Recovery week | AM: | Rest day | B L4, 60 mins into 20 mins R off **B** L1 | S L2, 45 mins | B L3, 45 mins | Rest day | S L1/2, 90 mins | Rest day | c.7 hrs |
| | PM: | | | R L3, 60 mins | S&C 30 mins | | R or **B** L3, 60 mins | | |
| 9 | AM: | S L2, 60 mins, **D** | B L2, 60 mins, **D** | S L2/3, 60 mins | B L3, 60 mins | Rest day | S L1/2, 90 mins | B L3, 120 mins | c.13 hrs |
| | PM: | R L2, 60 mins | S&C 30 mins | R L3, 60 mins | S&C 30 mins | | R L1/2, 150 mins | | |
| 10 | AM: | S L2, 45 min | B L2, 40 mins, **D** | S L4, 60 mins | B L3, 45 mins | Rest day | S L3, 90 mins | B L1, 330 mins into 10 mins R off **B** at race pace | c.13 hrs |
| | PM: | R L1, 30 mins easy recovery | S&C 30 mins | R L2, 90 mins | S&C 30 mins | | Rest | | |
| 11 | AM: | S L4, 60 mins | B L2, 45 mins, **D** | S L3, 60 mins | B L3, 60 mins | **START TAPER** ← | S L2, 75 mins | B L3, 90 mins into 40 mins R off **B** build from L1 to race pace | c.9 hrs |
| | PM: | R L1, 50mins | S&C 15 mins, trunk only | R L2, 60mins race pace work | S&C 10 mins, trunk only | Rest day | Rest | | |
| 12 Recovery week | AM: | S L3, 40 mins | B L2/3, 60 mins into 20 mins R off **B** L1 | S L3, 40 mins | B L2, 40 mins into 10 mins R off **B** L2 | Rest day | S pick ups L1-3, 20 mins  B pick ups L1-3, 20 mins  R pick ups L1-3 15 mins | **RACE DAY** **S** 3.8km **B** 180km **R** 42km | c.17 hrs |
| | PM: | | S&C 10 mins, trunk only | | Rest | | | | |

# KEEPING A TRAINING LOG

**Some athletes enjoy tracking** their training, while others find it a chore. Keeping a training log will give you a clear overview of your day-to-day progress. It will also help you analyse what you are doing well and where you need to improve.

*❝ AS RACE DAY LOOMS AND NERVES KICK IN, IT WILL BOOST YOUR CONFIDENCE TO LOOK BACK OVER YOUR TRAINING LOG AND SEE HOW MUCH YOU HAVE ACHIEVED AND HOW FAR YOU HAVE PROGRESSED. ❞*

### WHAT'S THE POINT OF A LOG?

**A** Keeping a log will help you track what has worked well for you during training. It will also help you identify factors that may have had a negative impact on your performance, such as a change in your waking heart rate, an injury, or a bad night's sleep. A training log can also be a great source of motivation – if you are feeling nervous or lacking in confidence as the race approaches, you can look back on what you have already achieved during your training and feel proud of how much progress you have made.

### WHAT MAKES A REALLY GOOD LOG?

**A** The more information you record, the better-informed your analysis will be. Set your data out in a clear format so that you can see everything at a glance. Once you have developed a system that works for you, use it consistently; it will save you time later when you need to compare data quickly. You also need to be honest with yourself – don't be tempted to cheat and record more than you actually did. If you had a bad day, use it to motivate yourself to work harder next time.

### WHAT SHOULD I INCLUDE?

**A** Ideally you should keep a record of each training session with details of your speed, heart rate, and level of exercise (see opposite). It's also a good idea to keep a daily record of your nutrition, sleep patterns, and general health as this may help you identify why you are feeling tired or lacking in motivation. Perhaps most importantly, try to record how you felt during the session. This will help you to identify what you did well and what you need to do to improve during your next sessions.

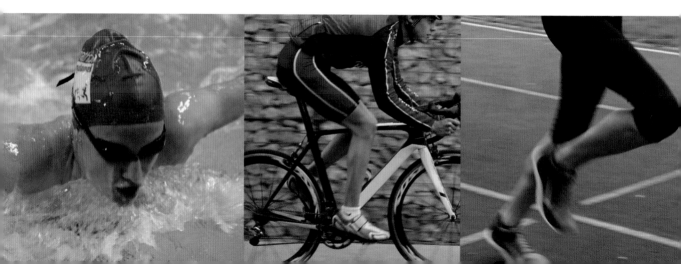

## HOW TO RECORD

There are numerous online training logs that you can use to record data from your workouts. If you are using a GPS watch (see p.32) you can upload data directly to the log.

If you don't have a GPS watch, you can record your pace using the measurements of your local pool or running track (or any space with a known measurement). You will have already worked out your average pace for each training zone during your profiling sessions (see p.118).

You can also check your heart rate manually by finding your pulse and counting the beats for 15 seconds and multiplying it by 4.

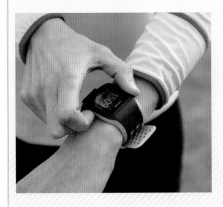

### WHAT TO RECORD PER SESSION

• **Time of day** Make a note of the times of your workouts. If you are cramming two sessions together, you may discover that your performance is suffering because you're not giving yourself enough time to recover. You may also find that you are performing better at certain times of the day.

• **Session details** Use your log to record details such as your speeds, distances, heart rate, power, and pace as well as the duration of the workout and the number of sets and repetitions you completed. Make a note of any factors that may have affected your performance, such as the weather, road conditions, or water temperature.

• **How you felt** It is useful to record your thoughts and feelings after a session. It will help you analyze your performance and work out whether factors such as stress or fatigue have had a negative impact on your training.

**GPS watch** Data such as heart rate and speed can be uploaded directly onto your computer, which will save you valuable time.

### WHAT TO RECORD PER DAY

• **Waking heart rate** Check your heart rate first thing in the morning as it is the best indicator of your overall health and well-being (see p.29).

• **Hours slept** An athlete training for a triathlon will need between 6 and 9 hours' sleep per night.

• **Sleep quality** The better you sleep, the more refreshed you will feel. Keep a record of your sleep patterns, so that you can spot problems as they emerge.

• **Fatigue levels** Prolonged muscle soreness, or feeling over-tired, can be a sign of Underperformance Syndrome (see pp.134-135).

• **Nutrition** Even a healthy diet may need adjusting, so it's useful to check whether what you have eaten has had an impact on your performance.

• **Hydration** Keep an eye on your hydration levels by checking the colour of your urine (see p.93).

• **Stress levels** It can be useful to recognize that stress caused by work, family, or other problems can lead to poor performance.

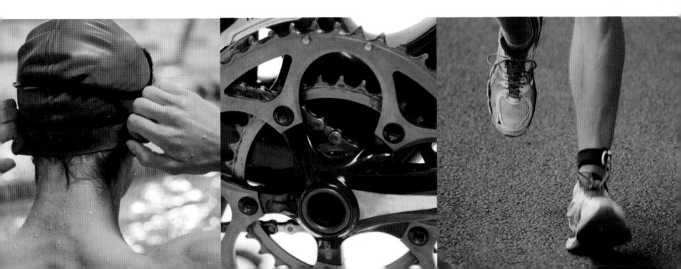

# AVOID OVERTRAINING AND UNDERPERFORMING

**When training for three disciplines,** as an athlete you need to be smart. You cannot just train, train, train – your approach has to be about the balance between training and recovery. Excessive training weakens the body, so if you overdo it, you'll end up undermining your performance.

> " A **HAPPY** ATHLETE IS A **STRONG** ATHLETE. IF YOU'RE TIRED AND DISCOURAGED, FOCUS ON **LOOKING AFTER YOURSELF.** "

## YOUR ROUTE TO SUCCESS

### UNDERPERFORMANCE

If you regularly look back over your training log (see pp.132–133), you should see a reasonably steady linear progression. But if it shows that your performance levels are static or getting worse, you may be overtraining. Training too hard or too often, allowing insufficient recovery time, and poor refuelling can result in underperformance. This may lead to a cycle of fatigue and poor performance known as Underperformance Syndrome. Overtraining also increases your risk of injury (see pp.154–157).

### FINDING THE CAUSES

Examine your training log for clues as to why you're underperforming. Maybe you did three big training days in a row without recovering properly between them? Or perhaps you increased your training volume more than 10 per cent but didn't add extra rest time? Emotional and psychological factors can also play a part. Are work problems, money difficulties, or relationship or family issues bothering you? Juggling all of life's commitments is hard enough without a triathlon to train for; if another area starts to dominate, your performance will suffer.

### HOW TO AVOID IT

Log your waking heart rate twice a week. An increase of more than 10–15 beats per minute indicates that your body's under stress. Make sure you're properly hydrated and nourished (see pp.88–93), so that what you eat and drink works with your body, not against it. Never neglect your recovery time.

Over-reaching – a short-term training overload – is fine if it's planned and well managed. For example, if you go to a camp or take a week's holiday to train, you can increase your training volume by several hours, provided that you factor in daytime naps and longer nights' sleep. Pay attention to how you feel. If you lack motivation and aren't enjoying training, that can be a sign you need more self-care.

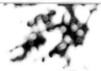

## THE TRAINING CURVE

Good effort generally leads to good progress. But sustained, unplanned, or poorly managed over-reaching (training beyond your peak) can push you into Underperformance Syndrome. At that point, listen to the messages your body is sending you and give it plenty of recovery time. Don't be afraid to miss training sessions – it will help your performance in the long term.

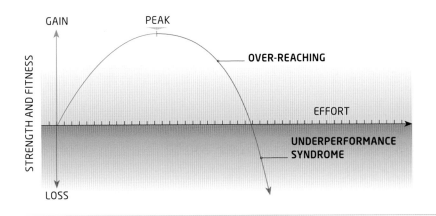

## GETTING BACK ON TRACK

If you're underperforming, don't respond by pushing yourself even harder. When performance levels drop, some people do extra training because they're worried they're not hitting their times, but this will just make things worse. Usually 48 hours' rest with plenty of sleep and good food will put you back on track. If it doesn't, see your doctor.

## SYMPTOMS TO WATCH FOR

Here are some of the typical symptoms of Underperformance Syndrome:

- Your performance is suffering despite all your efforts
- Chronic fatigue and lack of energy
- Persistent sore muscles and aching joints
- Trouble sleeping
- Frequent injuries
- Lack of appetite and decreasing body weight
- Frequent colds or respiratory infections
- Feeling higher levels of stress
- Elevated resting heart rate

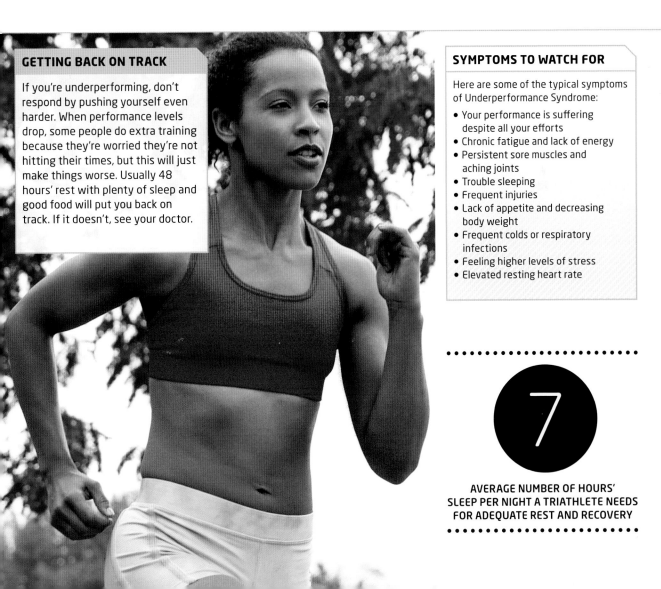

# 7

AVERAGE NUMBER OF HOURS'
SLEEP PER NIGHT A TRIATHLETE NEEDS
FOR ADEQUATE REST AND RECOVERY

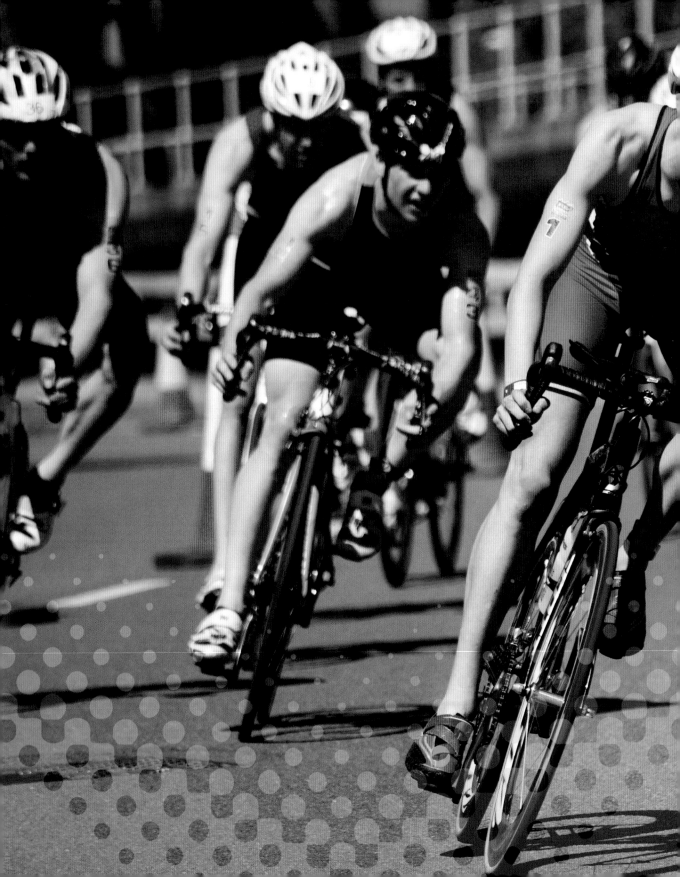

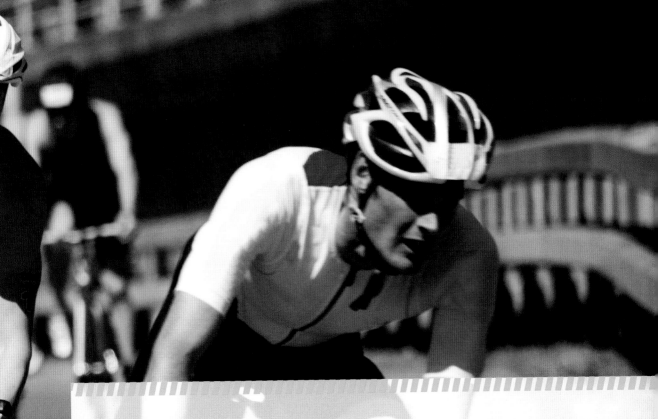

# THE RACE

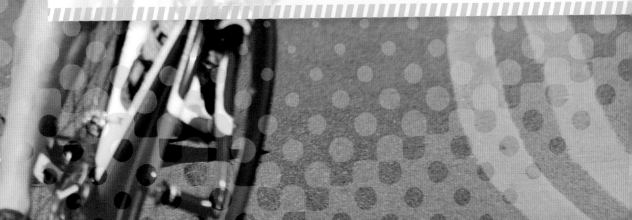

# TAPER YOUR TRAINING

**Training involves gradually** building up your effort levels, with the biggest volume of training a few weeks before your main event. However, if you enter the last few days of race preparation tired, you will not perform well; everyone benefits from easing off a little. How you taper (reduce) the volume of training and for how long depends on the individual. Whether it's a few days or weeks, tapering is a key part of your programme.

> **" CLIMB A FLIGHT OF STAIRS** A FEW DAYS BEFORE THE RACE. IF YOUR **LEGS START TO ACHE**, YOU NEED TO **TAPER SOME MORE. "**

## YOUR ROUTE TO SUCCESS

### TAPER TO YOUR PEAK

Tapering is a chance to freshen up mentally and physically. We build up fitness during recovery, so to get your body in peak condition for the race, you must give it extra time to recover. You won't stop exercising, but instead of pushing your fitness levels higher, you'll simply work to maintain them. This is also a time to focus on your nutrition. The aim is to let the muscles repair themselves and top up their stores of glycogen (carbohydrate), which will provide energy in the race (see pp.90–91). A good taper can help protect you from fatigue on race day and reduce the risk of injury.

### REDUCE TRAINING VOLUME

When tapering, your training volume should fall overall to 40-60 per cent of your last full-on week. As a rough guide, lower it by 20 per cent per week if you are on a three-week taper, and by 30 per cent per week for a two-week taper. If you are only tapering for 10 days, train at 50 per cent volume for the whole period. Don't worry about losing condition: tapering is too brief for that to happen.

### WATCH THE CALORIES

You may want to eat a little bit less during tapering. Taking in the same amount of calories as normal can leave you feeling bloated and heavy. Muscles can store only so much glycogen. Once they're at full capacity, excess calories will get stored as fat, which won't help your race preparations. Now is not the time to diet, though, because you don't want to weaken yourself. Adjust your eating regime to what feels comfortable, and keep a close eye on how your body responds.

# THREE-WEEK TAPER

During tapering, try to exercise at your normal times and keep to the same intensity, but reduce the overall duration of sessions. If you are tired and want to skip a session, do so.

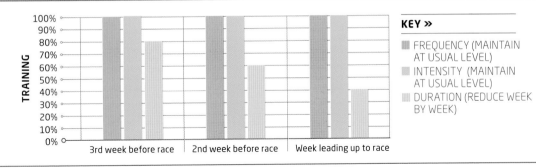

TRAINING

100%
90%
80%
70%
60%
50%
40%
30%
20%
10%
0%

3rd week before race    2nd week before race    Week leading up to race

**KEY »**

- FREQUENCY (MAINTAIN AT USUAL LEVEL)
- INTENSITY (MAINTAIN AT USUAL LEVEL)
- DURATION (REDUCE WEEK BY WEEK)

## AEROBIC BENEFITS

Tapering is excellent for your aerobic efficiency. Studies indicate that a healthy tapering pattern improves your red blood cell size and also increases your levels of haemoglobin – the protein that carries oxygen in the blood. This means that, come race day, your body will be primed to transport oxygen to your muscles so they can release all that stored energy (see pp.120–121). In the final few days of a taper, you should feel energized, full of motivation, and ready to go.

# PRE-RACE PREPARATION

**It is normal for triathletes** to feel nervous before a race. Anxiety causes the body to produce adrenaline, which increases your heart rate and can leave you feeling weak. The key is to use your nervous energy to boost your performance. If you can control your anxiety, you are more likely to perform well.

> " MANY ATHLETES **DON'T SLEEP WELL** BEFORE A BIG EVENT. THIS IS PERFECTLY NORMAL. TRY TO HAVE AN **EARLY NIGHT** TWO DAYS BEFORE THE RACE INSTEAD. "

## Q HOW CAN I FEEL CONFIDENT?

**A** Your mental preparation can be more important than your physical one, so you should try to approach every race with a positive attitude. Remind yourself that you have trained hard and are in great physical shape. Good preparation is key – you will feel more confident knowing that you have checked your equipment, fuelled your body efficiently, and done your pre-race rehearsal. Visualizing positive movement patterns for the swim, bike, and run sections will give you a great physical and mental boost.

## Q HOW DO I KEEP MY NERVE?

**A** You need to feel rested and relaxed to perform well, so try not to focus on negative thoughts or get over-exhausted before a race. Make sure you get enough sleep in the weeks prior to the race, and if you feel yourself becoming too anxious, try to distract yourself by doing other things such as seeing friends.

## Q HOW DO I STAY FOCUSED?

**A** As race day approaches, it is important not to lose your concentration. Plan as much as you can in advance: leaving everything until the last minute causes stress and will increase your chances of forgetting something important. Create a checklist of essential equipment (see opposite) and start putting everything together a few days in advance. Go over your race strategy, check your registration details, and get to the course in good time. If you live more than two hours away, it is a good idea to stay nearby the night before.

## Q CAN I MAKE LAST-MINUTE CHANGES?

**A** If you are feeling confident in the run-up to the race, it is tempting to over-inflate your race plan. Similarly, if your confidence drops, you might panic and feel the need to make last-minute changes. This is why it's important to set your race strategy ahead of race week – and stick to it. It's not a good idea to break in new trainers or try a new food just before the race. If a piece of kit breaks then obviously you will need to repair or replace it, but last-minute changes are more likely to undermine your performance than help it.

## Q CAN I PREPARE FOR THE UNEXPECTED?

**A** There will be elements of the triathlon that are beyond your control – such as the weather. As you become more experienced, you will encounter a variety of different race scenarios. It's a good idea to think about the kinds of things that might go wrong and work out a plan in advance. Set yourself race goals that focus on elements you can control, such as your pace and target finish time. These goals will help you to stay focused and motivated during the race. If unexpected events do occur, be ready to adapt. Above all, don't dwell on the negatives; focus on the present and visualize yourself crossing the finishing line.

## RESEARCH THE COURSE

Make sure you are familiar with the course before the race. Some triathlon websites offer aerial photos; if not, look at a map or view the location online. If possible, visit the site beforehand to get an idea of the terrain and conditions. If you have time, it's a good idea to drive the course and look for key landmarks: these will give you a sense of progression on the day.

## WHAT TO CHECK

Limit your kit to essential items and practise laying it out the night before.

### Warm up
- Spare trainers to warm up in
- Warming oil (if conditions are cold)
- Sports clothing to warm up in
- Waterproofs (if raining)

### Swim
- Swim hat
- Goggles (at least 2 pairs)
- Wetsuit (if using)
- Tri suit
- GPS watch
- Transition towel

### Bike
- Bike
- Helmet
- Cycling shorts/top (or tri suit)
- Sunglasses
- Race belt
- Cycling shoes (and elastic bands)
- Spare inner tubes
- Bike pump and puncture kit
- Bike computer/power meter
- Water bottle

### Run
- Running shoes
- Running shorts/top (or tri suit)
- Socks (if you are wearing them)
- Hat (in hot weather)
- Nutrition for run

### Recovery
- Warm/comfortable clothes
- Comfortable shoes
- Recovery fuel

### ENROLMENT
Register and get your numbers, then go straight to transition to set up and familiarize yourself with the layout.

### PRE-RACE
Set out your kit in your transition area. Identify the quickest routes back to your area from the swim-in and bike-in.

### SWIM
Think about your start and tactics for the race. Double-check the best route back from the swim to your transition area.

### TRANSITION AREA

### BIKE
Check your gears, tyres, bike computer, and power meters. Attach your helmet, shoes, and water bottle to the bike.

### TRANSITION AREA

### RUN
Open your trainers as much as possible for ease of access. Make sure you have fuel for the run and a hat (if it's hot).

### FINISH
Have some cash to buy a treat and make sure your mobile phone is charged so you can let your loved ones know you made it.

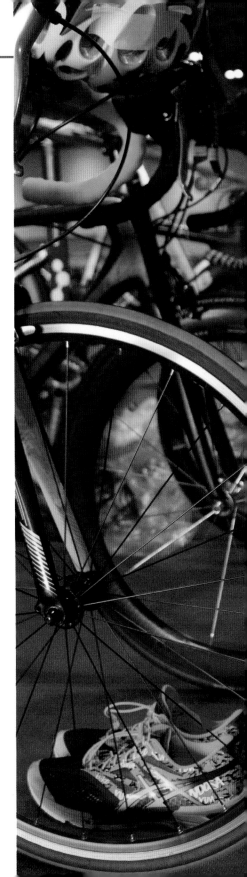

# FUEL YOUR PERFORMANCE

**When race day finally arrives**, you will need to be adequately fuelled. A triathlon pushes the body hard and burns up energy quickly. The amount of fuel you need depends on the duration of the race and the level of intensity at which you compete.

**"** A **BEGINNER TRIATHLETE** CAN TYPICALLY RACE FOR **90 MINUTES** WITHOUT NEEDING TO REFUEL. **EXPERIENCED ATHLETES** RACING AT A **HIGHER INTENSITY** MAY NEED TO REFUEL AFTER ABOUT **60 MINUTES**. **"**

## YOUR ROUTE TO SUCCESS

### HOW MANY CALORIES?

Knowing how many calories you burn at different levels of intensity will help you determine how much fuel you need during a race.

If you have been eating correctly and training efficiently at Levels 1 and 2 (see pp.160-161), your body will have learned to use fat stores for energy. A typical triathlete will have around 50,000 calories of stored fat, so should not need to refuel during low-intensity training.

If you have been training or racing at the higher intensities for more than 60 minutes, you will need to fuel your body. Current recommendations suggest 120-360 calories from carbohydrates per hour, but this can vary considerably from person to person.

During training, you should experiment with what works best for you. Using a GPS watch will give you an indication of how many calories you use at different levels of intensity.

### WHAT FOODS ARE BEST?

You should already be following a healthy, balanced diet while training (see pp.88-91). Two days before the race, start to increase your low-GI carbs for extra glycogen. Keep up your intake of fat and protein, and add small amounts of sea salt or rock salt to your diet (see pp.92-93) to balance your electrolytes (essential minerals in the blood that are lost through sweat). Avoid unfamiliar foods in the run-up to the race as they may upset your digestive system.

### WHAT SIZE PORTIONS?

As you approach race week, you will enter the tapering phase of your training (see pp.138-139). At this point you should cut out foods high in sugar and calories to avoid feeling bloated or heavy. However, do not cut down on healthy, nutritious food and do still eat whenever you feel hungry.

## TYPES OF FUEL

During exercise, your body's primary fuel source is carbohydrate, stored in the muscles as glycogen (see p.51). However, as you can only store a limited amount, you may need to refuel during longer or high-intensity races. Some athletes find energy gels, bars, and sports drinks helpful during a race, but whatever you choose, make sure that you trial it first in training so that you know it works for you.

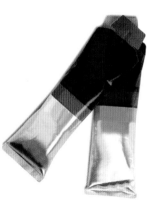

# WHEN TO EAT

Getting the right fuel means planning in advance: you want to avoid racing on a full stomach, but you also need to keep your energy levels up. If your triathlon starts in the morning, have a low-GI carbohydrate meal the night before to top up your glycogen levels.

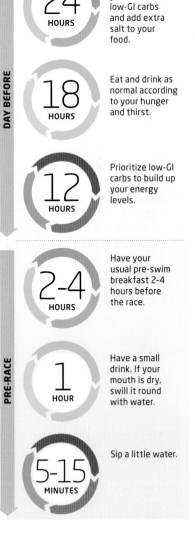

**DAY BEFORE**

**24 HOURS** — Eat and drink as usual. Increase your intake of low-GI carbs and add extra salt to your food.

**18 HOURS** — Eat and drink as normal according to your hunger and thirst.

**12 HOURS** — Prioritize low-GI carbs to build up your energy levels.

**PRE-RACE**

**2–4 HOURS** — Have your usual pre-swim breakfast 2–4 hours before the race.

**1 HOUR** — Have a small drink. If your mouth is dry, swill it round with water.

**5–15 MINUTES** — Sip a little water.

## HOW DO I TIME MY MEALS?

During training, you should eat little and often throughout the day. In the run-up to the race, stick to your regular meal times as a sudden change in eating patterns can confuse your digestive system. Avoid eating a large meal too close to the start of the race; if you race too soon after your main meal, it will weigh you down and you will feel heavy and sluggish.

## SHOULD I EAT AFTERWARDS?

After the race, you can eat whatever you feel like. You may want to reward yourself with a well-earned treat – perhaps something that you cut out of your pre-race diet. Don't worry too much about refuelling immediately after the race – the body will replace lost nutrients over the next day or so. If you can't face the thought of food after the race, don't force yourself to eat.

# HYDRATION TIPS

**When you race,** you sweat, and when you sweat, you lose water and body salts. Your training sessions will have helped you to work out how best to manage your hydration levels in different weather conditions and at different stages of the race, so use this information to stay hydrated on the day. Stick to what you know and you will avoid both under- and over-hydrating.

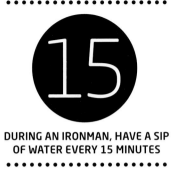

**15**

DURING AN IRONMAN, HAVE A SIP OF WATER EVERY 15 MINUTES

### BEFORE THE RACE

Before the race, you need to keep your fluid levels in a state of balance. Nerves can cause some athletes to take constant sips of water. This will not only make you want to urinate more frequently, it will also flush electrolytes (essential minerals in the blood) out of your system. Have some water if you are thirsty, but if you are drinking from nerves, swill your mouth with water and then spit it out.

### DURING THE RACE

If you are doing a longer race, such as Ironman or 70.3 (half Ironman), you need to be a little more systematic about when you fuel and drink. This is also the case if you are racing in hot or humid weather. You can stay hydrated with water – there will be plenty of water stations along the route – but you may also want to add a little sea or rock salt to your water bottle before the race, in order to replace the electrolytes lost in sweat. The amount you sweat will vary depending on the weather conditions and the

intensity and duration of the race. In shorter races, just drink when you are thirsty, but remember, don't drink too much as excess liquid sloshing about in your system can make you feel uncomfortable.

### AFTER THE RACE

If you are thirsty after the race, drink whatever you feel like – you will replace any nutrients lost in sweat over

time. If the race has been intense, some people like to have a hypertonic sports drink (see p.92). These have a high concentration of carbohydrates, and while you shouldn't drink them before or during a race (as they can interfere with electrolyte and fluid absorption during exercise), they can be a useful way to help you recover afterwards. Others just want a warm cup of tea!

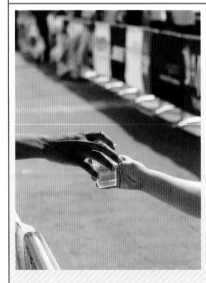

### TOO LITTLE OR TOO MUCH?

It's very rare for people to dehydrate during triathlons as there are normally water stations every few kilometres. Dehydration causes your blood to thicken; this makes it harder for your heart to work efficiently, and your cells end up getting less oxygen.

Overdrinking is a much more common problem in endurance events, especially among athletes towards the back of the race. Overdrinking during an event can cause the normal levels of sodium in the blood to drop. Very low sodium levels are dangerous and can result in seizures and coma. That said, these outcomes are very unlikely if you plan a good hydration strategy, so there's no need to panic.

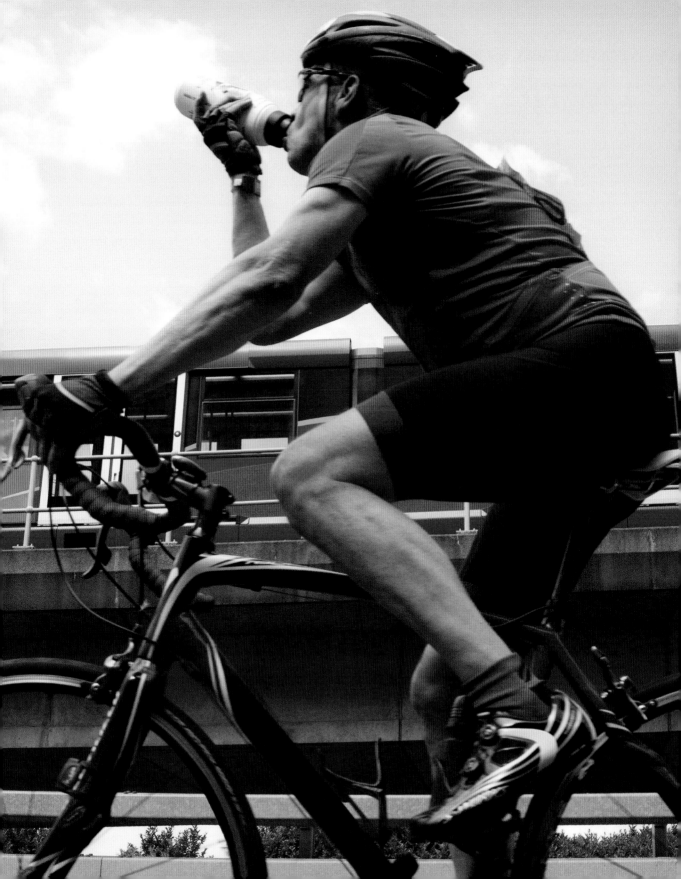

# TACTICS FOR RACE DAY

**When you reach the starting line,** you should be raring to go and buzzing with energy after a good taper (see pp.138-139), though it is natural to have butterflies. Remember that this is an endurance race: one common mistake is to start too fast, so think about your pacing strategy for the whole event.

**❝ RESPECT YOUR RACE PACE.** YOU'RE NOT IN A TRIATHLON TO BEAT OTHER PEOPLE, BUT TO **GIVE THE BEST PERFORMANCE** YOU CAN – AND THAT MEANS **SUSTAINABLE PACING. ❞**

## YOUR ROUTE TO SUCCESS

### PLAN YOUR TRANSITIONS

One thing you can only do on race day is familiarize yourself with the transition area and set up your gear there. Transition can be chaotic, and if you aren't exactly sure where everything is you may lose valuable minutes searching - minutes that you took months to save during your fitness training. A little bit of planning will make your transitions go smoothly (see pp.34-35, 56-57).

### SWIM PACE

In this leg, you won't be able to check your GPS watch or see if you are on target pace, but you'll know from your training (see pp.26-27) what your sustainable race pace feels like. It is good practice to "draft" a fellow competitor who swims at a slightly faster pace than you. This involves swimming in their slipstream to save energy. Sight the buoys at least every six strokes; it may feel like a hassle, but you'll lose less time than if you stray off course and add unnecessary metres to your swim (see pp.30-31).

### BIKE PACE

A power meter is the best device to monitor how you are doing on the bike leg. If you don't have a power meter, a heart-rate monitor is next best; failing that, be acutely aware of your RPE. Resist the urge to go with faster riders, and keep to your race pace or you will end up having to walk on the run. During training (see pp.48-49), you'll have planned how long each sector or kilometre should take, but now you will be cycling with others around you, which may affect your timings.

## RACE-DAY CHECKLIST

Come race day, you will have trained hard for a number of weeks, and learned many new skills and techniques, so don't risk ruining it all by forgetting the basics. Make a checklist of the essential things you need to do - and should avoid - to ensure you perform at your best.

**DON'T**

- Forget to check the course beforehand
- Forget to listen to the race briefing (things may change at the last minute)
- Forget sighting buoys during the swim - it's key to keeping you in your race
- Forget to pace yourself in all three disciplines
- Ever let negative thoughts beat you

**DO**

- Plan your race strategy in advance
- Know your transition area (both in and out)
- Make sure you have tested all your kit
- Start the swim in the right place for you
- Keep to your race pace in every discipline
- Save something for the sprint finish
- Believe in yourself

### RUN PACE

When you come off the bike you'll have jelly legs for a while. How long they last depends on your training and experience, and how hard you pushed yourself during the ride. Don't be discouraged: your running legs will come back. Use your heart-rate monitor and GPS watch to keep track of your run pace. Aim to maintain your race pace (don't speed up) even if you are feeling good, as you never know when things will get tough. If you're feeling tired, recall your training sessions (see pp.76-77) and focus on your technique.

### NO-MAN'S LAND

During your triathlon - especially in the run - you're likely to go through phases that are particularly tough. When this happens - typically about halfway through a discipline - it's described as being in "no-man's land". This is the key test of endurance and you need to work hard mentally to get through it. Visualize those times in training and in B races when you felt strong and confident, and be proud of yourself when you master this tricky section of triathlon racing. Your pre-race preparation (see pp.140-141) will have equipped you with enough mental tools to see you through.

### FINISH STRONG

Even if you have paced yourself perfectly, you will feel exhausted towards the end of the race. You may start to think too much about where the finish line is. If this happens, stay strong and concentrate on the present. Only when you see the finish line, or if a competitor is trying to sprint past you at the end, should you think about picking up the pace.

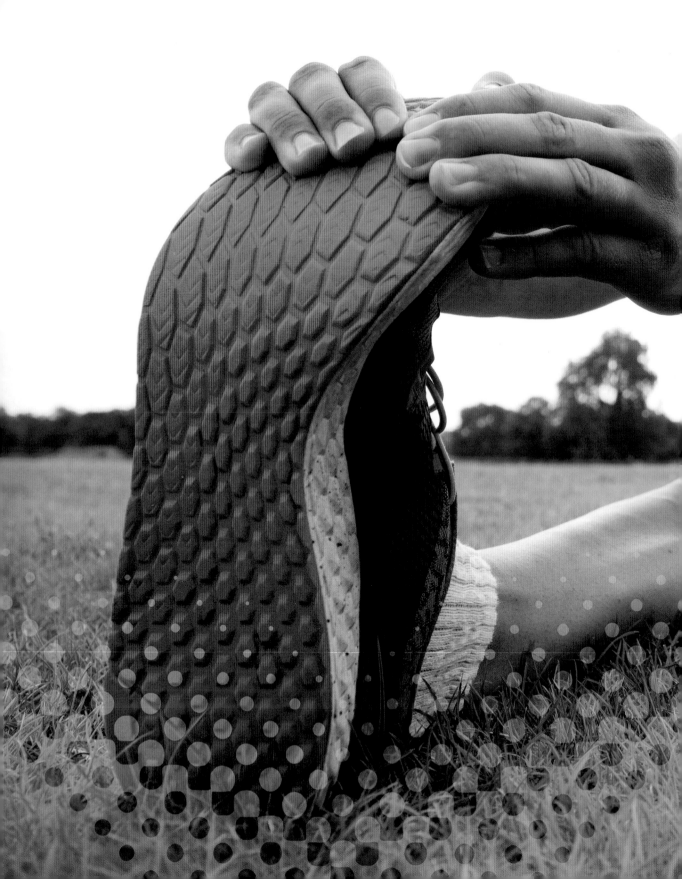

# ESSENTIAL MAINTENANCE

# PRE-HAB

**Pre-habilitation is a series** of exercises aimed at reducing the risk of injury. The triathlon regime is intensive; elite female athletes train for 25-30 hours a week, and elite male athletes for 35-40 hours. The foam-roller exercises below can be used all year round and are designed to keep soft tissue healthy.

## PRE-HAB EQUIPMENT

A foam roller is a firm cylinder - you lie on it and "roll" to massage areas of muscle tightness. It can be uncomfortable at first, but becomes easier as the soft tissue becomes healthier. For localized areas, try applying gradual pressure with a tennis or golf ball to ease the tension.

### FOAM ROLLER TIPS

- Start with a softer, low-density foam roller and progress from there
- Don't over-use the roller after strenuous sessions, as the muscle tissues need time to heal
- Use the roller on recovery days or after lighter workouts
- Try to roll upwards, towards the heart, to avoid over-straining vein valves
- Pause on any sensitive spots and let the pressure ease the tightness
- Always treat both sides of the body
- Be careful around joints: roll over ligaments and tendons, but avoid rolling over bony areas
- Keep a relaxed breathing rhythm

## 01 UPPER AND LOWER BACK

This exercise reduces tightness in the muscles of your thoracic and lumbar spine. It helps with posture and breathing, and minimizes the risk of back pain for triathletes.

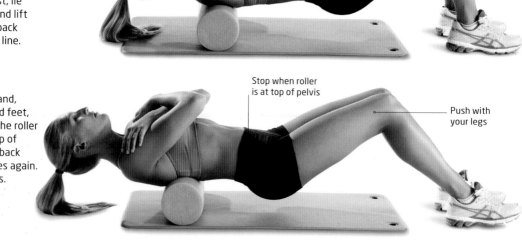

Feet should be slightly apart

Keep spine neutral

Raise hips off the floor

1 Sit down with knees bent and feet on the floor. Position the roller so that it is level with your shoulder blades. Place your arms across your chest, lie back onto the roller, and lift your hips. Keep your back and neck in a straight line.

Stop when roller is at top of pelvis

Push with your legs

2 Breathe normally and, using your legs and feet, push your body over the roller until it reaches the top of the pelvis, then work back to your shoulder blades again. Repeat for 30 seconds.

# 02 GLUTEAL AND PIRIFORMIS MUSCLES

This exercise focuses on the gluteal and piriformis muscles on the outer side of your buttocks. These muscles help with hip and leg stability and can over-tighten after running and cycling.

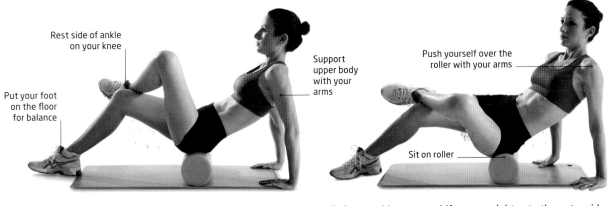

Rest side of ankle on your knee

Put your foot on the floor for balance

Support upper body with your arms

Push yourself over the roller with your arms

Sit on roller

1 Sit on the foam roller with your left buttock and cross your left leg over your right leg. Push your buttock backwards and forwards over the roller for 30 seconds. Sit on your right buttock, cross your legs, and repeat.

2 Rotate sideways to shift your weight onto the outer side of your left buttock. Cross your left leg over the right and push backwards and forwards over the roller. Turn to sit on the outer side of the right buttock, cross your legs, and repeat.

# 03 TFL MUSCLE AND ITB BAND

This exercise loosens the tensor fasciae latae (TFL) muscle of the upper leg and the iliotibial band (ITB), a band of fibrous tissue on the outer side of the leg. Runners and cyclists are especially prone to tightness in this area.

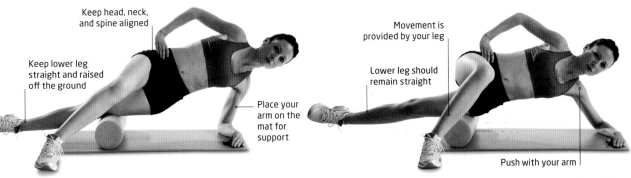

Keep head, neck, and spine aligned

Keep lower leg straight and raised off the ground

Place your arm on the mat for support

Movement is provided by your leg

Lower leg should remain straight

Push with your arm

1 Lie on your left side with the roller just above your knee. Support your upper body on your left forearm and place the other hand on your hip. Cross your right leg over the left, and put your right foot flat on the floor.

2 Using your left arm, gently push down over the roller until it is level with the top of your thigh, then pull back up until it is above your knee again. Repeat for 30 seconds. Turn over and repeat the exercise on your right leg.

# 04 HAMSTRING MUSCLES

This exercise helps to reduce muscle tension and imbalances in the hamstring muscles at the back of the thigh. Tension here is common in runners who actively use their hamstrings to run well.

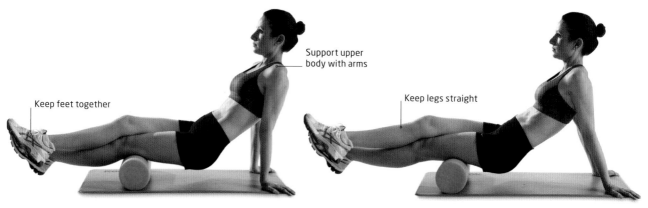

Support upper body with arms

Keep feet together

Keep legs straight

**1** Sit with your legs straight out in front and place the roller under the back of your knee. Cross your right leg over the left one at the knees. Raise your buttocks off the mat, keeping your head, neck, and spine aligned.

**2** Using your arms, push yourself over the roller, working from your knee to the base of your buttocks, then back to the knee. Repeat for at least 30 seconds. Cross your left leg over the right and repeat the exercise on your right leg.

# 05 QUADRICEPS MUSCLES

This exercise helps to reduce muscle tightness and imbalance at the front of the thighs. These muscles become tight due to repetitive muscle contraction, especially during a long run or swim. Tightness in these muscles can also affect your knees.

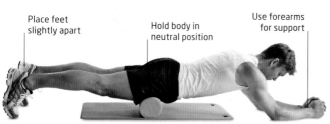

Place feet slightly apart

Hold body in neutral position

Use forearms for support

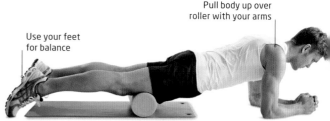

Use your feet for balance

Pull body up over roller with your arms

**1** Lie on your front with the roller beneath the top of your thighs. Keep your head, neck, body, and legs aligned. Support your upper body with your arms and make sure your toes are on the ground to support your legs.

**2** Move your body up until the roller is just above the knees, then work back to the top of the thighs (try to go right into the hip-flexor area). Repeat for 30 seconds. Crossing your legs at the ankles adds extra pressure, but always repeat on each leg.

# 06 **GASTROCNEMIUS** AND **SOLEUS** MUSCLES

This exercise reduces tension in the calf muscles and helps ankle mobility.
It is particularly helpful for cyclists and runners. Tightness in these muscles
can lead to pain in the Achilles tendon, heel, or foot arch.

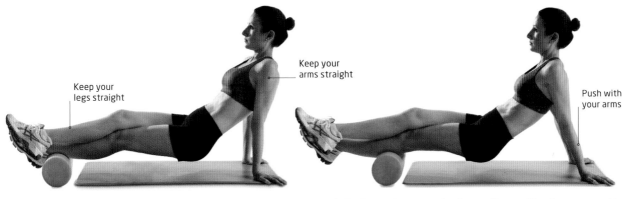

Keep your
arms straight

Keep your
legs straight

Push with
your arms

1 Sit with your legs straight, cross your right leg over the left,
and place the roller under the back of your ankles. Support
your upper body with your arms and lift your hips off the mat.

2 Push your legs over the foam roller, working from your ankle
to the back of the knee and back to the ankle again; repeat
for 30 seconds. Cross your left leg over the right leg and repeat
the exercise on your right leg.

# 07 **PLANTAR FASCIA** BAND

The plantar fascia is a band of tissue that supports the arch of the foot. It is
particularly prone to tension from repetitive stress caused by running long
distances. Using a golf ball helps to target smaller points of tension.

1 Sit down with your foot flat on
the floor, or stand up and hold
onto a chair back. Place a golf ball
on the floor and rest your foot on it.

2 Roll your foot over the golf ball, working in
a straight line from the ball of your foot to
the heel and back again. Increase the pressure
through your foot as required. Repeat the
exercise with your other foot.

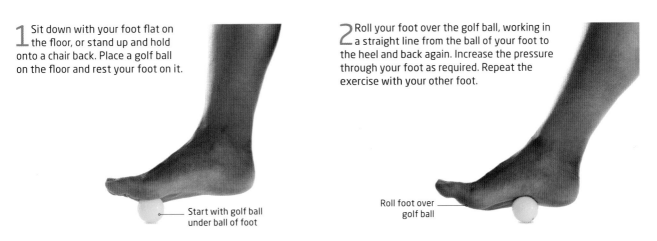

Start with golf ball
under ball of foot

Roll foot over
golf ball

# COMMON COMPLAINTS

**Most triathletes experience** a number of common complaints during training and racing. These are usually minor and can be prevented by a good pre-hab routine and regular massage (see pp.150-153). Most of the complaints listed below can be treated at home.

" AS YOU ARE DOING **THREE DYNAMIC SPORTS**, IT IS WORTH CONSIDERING DOING A **FIRST-AID COURSE**. THIS WILL GIVE YOU CONFIDENCE AS YOU ARE OUT THERE GETTING **FIT** AND **STRONG**. "

| COMPLAINT | PREVENTION | FIRST AID |
|---|---|---|
| **SWIMMER'S SHOULDER**<br>Pain in the shoulder can be caused by poor technique. It is normally due to the swimmer pulling too soon before the catch has been set up correctly (see the swimming drills on pp.20-27). | Ask a swimming coach to look at your technique. Make sure you use a variety of strokes to balance out the muscles used. Set up your catch properly (see pp.16-17 and 20-27). | Use massage and friction on the shoulder. Heat the area either with hot water in the shower or with a heat pad. If the problem persists, consult a physiotherapist. |
| **IRRITABLE NOSE**<br>Chlorine in the pool can irritate the lining of the nose. Runners and cyclists may suffer from a runny nose when training outside. This can be caused by allergies (such as hay fever) or by rhinitis (an inflammation of the nasal membranes). | Swim with a nose clip and use a low-chlorine pool. Use soft tissues (containing a soothing balm) to avoid chafing the skin. | Use a steam room to help to counteract the effects of chlorine. Runners and cyclists should seek medical advice if the nasal lining becomes inflamed. |
| **SADDLE SORES**<br>These are painful lesions on areas of skin that are in contact with the saddle (such as the buttocks, upper thighs, and groin). They are normally caused when the hair follicles become infected. | Use an antibacterial chamois cream which will reduce friction and help to avoid infection. Wash your cycling shorts frequently. | Wash the area with clean water and pat dry. Rub antiseptic cream onto the lesions. Visit your doctor if the area gets infected. |
| **ROAD RASH**<br>This is an area of painful grazing that occurs when a cyclist falls and makes contact with the road. Loss of skin can make clothing and sleeping uncomfortable. Affected areas may sting in the pool. | Lower the tyre pressure on your bike in wet conditions to improve your grip around corners. Keeping your legs shaved before you cycle will help to speed up healing. | Clean the area with warm soapy water to remove any road tar. Grazed areas will heal better if they are kept clean and dry. Avoid swimming until the area has healed. |
| **CARPAL TUNNEL SYNDROME**<br>This can occur after longer bike rides when the weight of the rider presses down through the hand. The nerve from the wrist to the hand becomes inflamed and sore. The usual symptoms are numbness in the hand and fingers. | Check the fit of your bike and make sure you don't overload the weight on your hands. Wear gloves with good padding around the problem nerve area. | Massaging the area helps to reduce numbness. Medically recommended exercises can also help. In very severe cases, surgery may be needed. |

| COMPLAINT | PREVENTION | FIRST AID |
|---|---|---|
| **BLISTERS**<br>Painful, fluid-filled blisters are caused by wearing unsuitable socks or training shoes that pinch, rub, or compress your feet. Blisters are not serious unless they become infected, but they can prevent you from training. | Ensure you wear well-fitting shoes and socks. Reduce friction by wearing double-skinned socks, and apply petroleum jelly or skin plasters. | You can run with a blister as long as it's not too painful. If the blister breaks, you will need to keep it clean or it may become infected. |
| **RUNNER'S TOE**<br>Bleeding under the toenail can create a black-looking toenail. It is caused by wearing ill-fitting footwear that puts pressure on the nail bed. Runner's toe is not usually serious, but it can be very painful. | Make sure your training shoes fit properly. Trim your toenails and check that you are not scuffing your foot into the ground when running. | If it is painful, stop running for a few days and keep the toe clean and dry to avoid infection. The nail may eventually drop off but it should soon grow back. |
| **LOWER-BACK PAIN**<br>This is not uncommon in triathletes and can have a number of causes. Most cases of lower-back pain are caused by injuries and overstraining in the lumbar region. It is more common in older triathletes and those who work at a desk. See also Sciatica on p.157. | Keep your back supple by doing regular mobility exercises. In the pool, use front scull and deep kick drills to avoid straining your back muscles. | Massage the affected area and stretch the muscles. Heat pads may also help. Stay active rather than resting, as movement will help to loosen tight muscles. |
| **DOMS**<br>Delayed onset muscle soreness (DOMS) is pain caused by micro-tearing of the muscle fibres during long or intensive exercise. It usually develops 12-24 hours after exercise, depending on the intensity of the workout. | Although DOMS cannot really be prevented if you want to overload your training, avoid progressing too quickly. Stretches will exacerbate it, so use flushing (see pp.69. 74-75). | Keep the area active and resume normal training as this is only a minor trauma to the body. Try increasing the protein levels in your diet for a few days (see pp.88-91). |
| **CRAMP**<br>The causes of cramp are largely unknown. It can occur in the muscles, or as a "stitch" in the side of the stomach. You can run through a stitch, but it is not advisable to keep running on a cramp in the muscle. | You can reduce your chance of cramp by making sure your electrolyte balance is good (see p.92) and keeping your muscles strong and supple. | Stop and rest for a while until the discomfort passes. Stretching and massage can also help. If the pain persists, seek medical advice. |
| **SUNBURN**<br>Exposure to the sun's ultraviolet (UV) rays can cause the skin to redden and peel (even in mild or overcast weather). Severe sunburn can be painful and may cause blisters. | Apply a high-factor sunscreen to exposed areas of skin, and wear protective clothing and sunglasses. Where possible, train in the shade. | Commercial after-sun creams can be helpful, as can cool water. Cover the burned area to avoid further damage. In severe cases, seek medical advice. |
| **HEAT-RELATED ILLNESS**<br>Overheating can lead to heat exhaustion, which causes dizziness, headaches, and cramps. In extreme cases this can lead to heatstroke, a life-threatening medical emergency in which the body's thermostat system fails altogether. | Make sure you are wearing appropriate clothing for hot weather. Increase your electrolyte intake (see p.92) and keep well hydrated. | Stay in the shade, keep cool, and make sure you do not drink too much too quickly (take small sips). In severe cases seek urgent medical advice. |

# COMMON INJURIES

**Almost every athlete** experiences injuries from time to time. Acute injuries, such as ruptured ligaments or torn muscles, can occur suddenly. Chronic injuries are caused by overuse and develop over time. It is important not to neglect injuries as they may develop into long-term problems if left untreated.

## USING ICE

Most soft-tissue injuries are minor and can be treated at home. Current medical guidelines recommend applying an ice pack (wrapped in a towel) to the area, while keeping the area raised and under compression for 20-30 minutes every two hours for the first three days. Over-icing, however, can limit the flow of healing blood cells to the area, and should be avoided.

### SOFT-TISSUE INJURIES

In the case of injuries to muscles, tendons, and ligaments:
- Stop activity immediately and assess the seriousness of the injury
- If the area is very painful, use ice and a compression bandage on the area, and keep the body part elevated
- If the pain or injury is severe, then seek urgent medical advice - if you cannot move, call an ambulance
- If it is not severe, then leave the injury for 48 hours, seeking medical advice if pain persists
- If there is no pain, then keep the affected area mobile and apply heat

| INJURY | SYMPTOMS | TREATMENT |
|---|---|---|
| **STRAIN** A strain is a pull, twist, or tear to a muscle, ligament, or tendon. There are three grades of strain: grade one is a mild tear; grade two is more serious, requiring complete recovery before training is resumed. For grade three, see below. | Pain, swelling, reduced movement, and possible redness. The pain can get worse when you exercise or put pressure on the area. | Use ice on the area if it's painful and try to keep it mobile (but do not put weight on it). Avoid pain-relief medication, as it can mask the pain and worsen the injury. |
| **SPRAIN** A sprain occurs when a ligament has been pulled, twisted, or torn. There are three grades of sprain: grade one is a minor injury; grade two needs full recovery before resuming training. For grade three, see below. | Pain, stiffness, and possible swelling. You may find it difficult to move the affected area or put weight on it. | Apply ice to the area if it is very painful. Avoid taking pain-relief medication as this can mask the pain and potentially result in further damage. |
| **GRADE THREE STRAIN OR SPRAIN** A grade-three strain or sprain is a total rupture or breakage of a muscle or tendon, or a ligament. Left untreated, it can result in permanent damage to the affected area and the formation of scar tissue. | Severe pain, swelling, reduced movement, and possible redness. You may also hear a "popping'" sound at the moment of injury. | Stop exercise immediately and seek medical advice. A complete rupture is likely to need surgery, followed by several weeks of physiotherapy. |
| **STRESS FRACTURES** These are small cracks in a bone (usually in the feet, legs, and pelvis) that can be caused by overuse, incorrect technique, or poor diet (see pp.88-91). Left untreated, they can develop into more serious fractures. | Localized tenderness (often on one side due to uneven balance). The area may feel hot and swollen, and you may be unable to put weight on it. | Cease exercise and seek medical advice. You may need an X-ray. Use non-weight-bearing exercise (under professional guidance) to stay fit. |
| **PATELLOFEMORAL PAIN SYNDROME** This is pain around the front of the knee (often resulting from earlier damage such as a fall), which can occur when your kneecap (patella) is affected by imbalances in the quadriceps muscles surrounding the knee. | Pain in the front of the knee, often when walking downstairs or running downhill. There may be a grating sensation within the joint (known as "crepitus"). | Stop activities that cause pain and use ice for pain relief. Consult a physiotherapist for exercises that will help the quad muscles realign the patella. |

| INJURY | SYMPTOMS | TREATMENT |
|---|---|---|
| **ACHILLES RUPTURE**<br>The feet and ankles are particularly susceptible to tendon injuries. Ruptures of the Achilles tendon may be partial but are more commonly complete. You are at greater risk of the injury occuring if you have a poor running technique, or have previously had Achilles tendinopathy (see below). | A sudden, usually intense pain in the calf, followed by varying degrees of bruising and swelling, and stiffness in the area. You may also hear an audible "snap" as the tendon tears. | Stop exercise immediately and seek medical attention. A complete rupture is likely to need surgery, followed by several weeks of physiotherapy. |
| **ACHILLES TENDINOPATHY**<br>This is a degerative condition caused by repetitive stress on the leg and ankle that is characterized by pain and inflammation in and around the Achilles tendon. While the condition is treatable, it is likely to reoccur in the future. Achilles tendinopathy is more common in older athletes. | Pain or discomfort around the Achilles tendon, sometimes accompanied by swelling and thickening around your tendon, and stiffness in your calf, especially just after waking up. | Rest, ice, and physiotherapy may help. If the condition doesn't improve, your doctor may refer you for an ultrasound or MRI scan. Severe cases may require surgery and rehabilitation. |
| **ILIOTIBIAL BAND SYNDROME (ITB)**<br>The ITB is a long tendon-like structure that extends down the upper leg from the hip to the outside of the knee. ITB syndrome occurs when the band becomes inflamed. Weak hip muscles, poor knee alignment, or overpronation (inward rolling) of the foot are common causes of the condition. | Pain on the outside of the knee when you bend or straighten it. The outer side of your upper leg may also feel painful, tight, or swollen. The condition may flare up after running. | Avoid running downhill or on a camber. Apply heat to the area and stop any activity that causes pain. Deep massage can be effective once the initial phase of acute pain has passed. |
| **PLANTAR FASCIITIS (HEEL SPUR PAIN)**<br>The arch ligament or plantar fascia is a fibrous band of tissue that runs from the heel to the toe. Pain occurs when too much load is put on the plantar fascia due to poor running technique (for example heel-striking). | Pain in the heel, particularly first thing in the morning, and numbness along the outside of the sole of the foot. The pain may disappear during periods of rest. | Keep immobilized until the pain stops. Consult a physiotherapist for advice on rehabilitation to strengthen your foot and correct your running technique. Resume training slowly. |
| **SHIN SPLINTS**<br>Technically known as "medial tibial periostitis", this condition is characterized by pain at the front of the shin. It is usually caused by an inadequate warm-up, a sudden increase in training, poor technique, running on hard surfaces, or running in unsuitable or worn-out footwear. | Pain on the inner side of the shin that often gets worse during exercise. Shin splints can be caused by compartment syndrome (see below). | Stop training and use heat or ice on the area until it is pain-free. Consult a physiotherapist to assess your running technique and discuss a strength-training rehabilitation routine. |
| **COMPARTMENT SYNDROME**<br>Muscles are contained within "compartments" of connective tissue and bone. Compartment syndrome is a painful swelling inside one such compartment that puts pressure on the nerves and blood vessels within. The condition can be caused by acute injury or by long-term overuse. | Pain which increases under weight-bearing load and makes continued exercise impossible. You may also experience a weakness, tingling, or slight numbness in the area. | Cease exercise and seek medical advice. Left untreated, compartment syndrome can cause permanent muscle and nerve damage. Surgery may be needed in severe cases. |
| **SCIATICA/SLIPPED DISC**<br>Back pain is common in runners and can have numerous causes, including poor technique. Pain that radiates from the back down to the leg is known as sciatica. One of the common causes of this is a slipped (prolapsed) disc, which exerts pressure on one of the roots of the sciatic nerve. | Stiffness and pain in the lower back (lumbar region). Sciatica can cause "pins and needles", numbness, and weakness in the legs, while a slipped disc may cause shooting pains. | Stop training, but try to stay mobile (if it is not too painful) to stop the muscles seizing up. Apply ice and take pain-relief medication, and seek medical advice if the symptoms persist. |

# FITNESS CHARTS

**Check these charts** to assess your fitness levels using the instructions on pp.29 and 79. The Cooper 12-minute test (opposite) is designed to calculate your VO2 max – your body's maximum capacity for oxygen intake.

**1,000**

NUMBER OF TIMES ITS OWN
WEIGHT THAT A MUSCLE
FIBRE CAN SUPPORT

## RESTING HEART RATE (P.29)

This is the simplest way of measuring your physical fitness – all you need is a watch or clock. Be careful not to move during the test; you can also test yourself at intervals throughout your training programme to see your progress.

» RESTING HEART RATES FOR MEN

| AGE | 18-25 | 26-35 | 36-45 | 46-55 | 56-65 | 65+ |
|---|---|---|---|---|---|---|
| ATHLETE | 49-55 | 49-54 | 50-56 | 50-57 | 51-56 | 50-55 |
| EXCELLENT | 56-61 | 55-61 | 57-62 | 58-63 | 57-61 | 56-61 |
| GOOD | 62-65 | 62-65 | 63-66 | 64-67 | 62-67 | 62-65 |
| ABOVE AVERAGE | 66-69 | 66-70 | 67-70 | 68-71 | 68-71 | 66-69 |
| AVERAGE | 70-73 | 71-74 | 71-75 | 72-76 | 72-75 | 70-73 |
| BELOW AVERAGE | 74-81 | 75-81 | 76-82 | 77-83 | 76-81 | 74-79 |
| POOR | 82+ | 82+ | 83+ | 84+ | 82+ | 80+ |

» RESTING HEART RATES FOR WOMEN

| AGE | 18-25 | 26-35 | 36-45 | 46-55 | 56-65 | 65+ |
|---|---|---|---|---|---|---|
| ATHLETE | 54-60 | 54-49 | 54-59 | 54-60 | 54-59 | 54-59 |
| EXCELLENT | 61-65 | 60-64 | 60-64 | 61-65 | 60-64 | 60-64 |
| GOOD | 66-69 | 65-68 | 65-69 | 66-69 | 65-68 | 65-68 |
| ABOVE AVERAGE | 70-73 | 69-72 | 70-73 | 70-73 | 69-73 | 69-72 |
| AVERAGE | 74-78 | 73-76 | 74-78 | 74-77 | 74-77 | 73-76 |
| BELOW AVERAGE | 79-84 | 77-82 | 79-84 | 78-83 | 78-83 | 77-84 |
| POOR | 85+ | 83+ | 85+ | 84+ | 84+ | 84+ |

## MAXIMAL OXYGEN UPTAKE (VO2 MAX) TESTING (P.79)

VO2 max is measured here in millilitres per kilogramme of body weight per minute (please note that in this book it is measured in metric units only). Use online calculators for your chosen test for a quick way of finding your score.

» RATING FOR MEN (ML/KG/MIN)

| AGE | 18-25 | 26-35 | 36-45 | 46-55 | 56-65 | 65+ |
|---|---|---|---|---|---|---|
| EXCELLENT | 60 | 56 | 51 | 45 | 41 | 37 |
| GOOD | 52-60 | 49-56 | 43-51 | 39-45 | 36-41 | 33-37 |
| ABOVE AVERAGE | 47-51 | 43-48 | 39-42 | 36-38 | 32-35 | 29-32 |
| AVERAGE | 42-46 | 40-42 | 35-38 | 32-35 | 30-31 | 26-28 |
| BELOW AVERAGE | 37-41 | 35-39 | 31-34 | 29-31 | 26-29 | 22-25 |
| POOR | 30-36 | 30-34 | 26-30 | 25-28 | 22-25 | 20-21 |
| VERY POOR | 30 | 30 | 26 | 25 | 22 | 20 |

» RATING FOR WOMEN (ML/KG/MIN)

| AGE | 18-25 | 26-35 | 36-45 | 46-55 | 56-65 | 65+ |
|---|---|---|---|---|---|---|
| EXCELLENT | 56 | 52 | 45 | 40 | 37 | 32 |
| GOOD | 47-56 | 45-52 | 38-45 | 34-40 | 32-37 | 28-32 |
| ABOVE AVERAGE | 42-46 | 39-44 | 34-37 | 31-33 | 28-31 | 25-27 |
| AVERAGE | 38-41 | 35-38 | 31-33 | 28-30 | 25-27 | 22-24 |
| BELOW AVERAGE | 33-37 | 31-34 | 27-30 | 25-27 | 22-24 | 19-21 |
| POOR | 28-32 | 26-30 | 22-26 | 20-24 | 18-21 | 17-18 |
| VERY POOR | 28 | 26 | 22 | 20 | 18 | 17 |

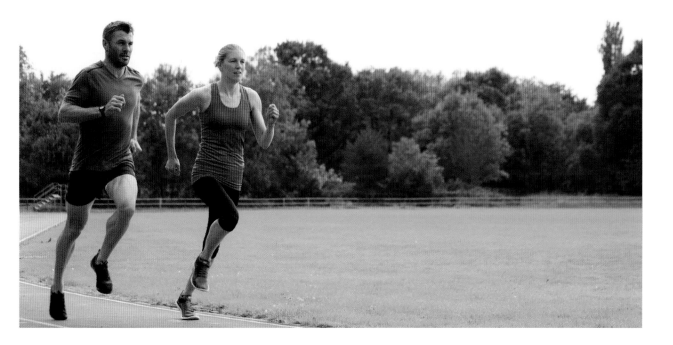

# THE COOPER 12-MINUTE TEST (P.79)

Perform this fitness test either on a running track or with a GPS watch – it simply involves running for 12 minutes and measuring the distance you cover. Correlate the results using the relevant equation on p.79 to find your VO2 max rating.

» RATING FOR MEN

| AGE | VERY GOOD | GOOD | AVERAGE | BAD | VERY BAD |
|---|---|---|---|---|---|
| 17-20 | 3,000+m (9,843+ft) | 2,700-3,000m (8,858-9,843ft) | 2,500-2,699m (8,202-8,857ft) | 2,300-2,499m (7,545-8,201ft) | 2,300-2,499m (7,545-8,201ft) |
| 20-29 | 2,800+m (9,186+ft) | 2,400-2,800m (7,874-9,186ft) | 2,200-2,399m (7,218-7,873ft) | 1,600-2,199m (5,249-7,217ft) | 1,600m (5,249ft) or less |
| 30-39 | 2,700+m (8,858+ft) | 2,300-2,700m (7,545-8,858ft) | 1,900-2,299m (6,234-7,544ft) | 1,500-1,899m (4,921-6,233ft) | 1,500m (4,921ft) or less |
| 40-49 | 2,500+m (8,202+ft) | 2,100-2,500m (6,890-8,202ft) | 1,700-2,099m (5,577-6,889ft) | 1,400-1,699m (4,593-5,576ft) | 1,400m (4,593ft) or less |
| 50+ | 2,400+m (7,874+ft) | 2,000-2,400m (6,562-7,874ft) | 1,600-1,999m (5,249-6,561ft) | 1,300-1,599m (4,265-5,248ft) | 1,300m (4,265ft) or less |

» RATING FOR WOMEN

| AGE | VERY GOOD | GOOD | AVERAGE | BAD | VERY BAD |
|---|---|---|---|---|---|
| 17-20 | 2,300+m (7,545+ft) | 2,100-2,300m (6,890-7,545ft) | 1,800-2,099m (5,905-6,889ft) | 1,700-1,799m (5,577-5,904ft) | 1,700m (5,577ft) or less |
| 20-29 | 2,700+m (8,858+ft) | 2,200-2,700m (7,218-8,858ft) | 1,800-2,199m (5,905-7,217ft) | 1,500-1,799m (4,921-5,904ft) | 1,500m (4,921ft) or less |
| 30-39 | 2,500+m (8,202+ft) | 2,000-2,500m (6,562-8,202ft) | 1,700-1,999m (5,577-6,561ft) | 1,400-1,699m (4,593-5,576ft) | 1,400m (4,593ft) or less |
| 40-49 | 2,300+m (7,545+ft) | 1,900-2,300m (6,234-7,545ft) | 1,500-1,899m (4,921-6,233ft) | 1,200-1,499m (3,937-4,920ft) | 1,200m (3,937ft) or less |
| 50+ | 2,200+m (7,218+ft) | 1,700-2,200m (5,577-7,218ft) | 1,400-1,699m (4,593-5,576ft) | 1,100-1,399m (3,609-4,592ft) | 1,100m (3,609ft) or less |

# TRAINING LEVELS

**Training for triathlon** requires varying levels of effort. Training levels are a way of measuring the intensity of this effort and monitoring your performance as you strive to achieve a given speed for the least possible effort. Each of the five levels has varying biological effects and offers different benefits, summarized here. Taking these as a guide, tailor your training to your race goals, and then go out and have fun as you swim, bike, and run.

## UNDERSTANDING TRAINING LEVELS

The chart on the right will help you to monitor the intensity of your training, and to know which level to aim for when competing. The levels are given as percentages of maximum heart rate (% of HR max), but they vary for different people. Most endurance athletes work on the 80:20 principle – 80 per cent of training is done at or around Levels 1 and 2, and 20 per cent is at or around Levels 3, 4, or 5.

### Aerobic exercise
Low-intensity exercise that enables your body to take in enough oxygen to combine with its stores of fat and glycogen to make fuel, producing lactate as a by-product.

### Anaerobic exercise
Exercise of such an intensity that your body cannot take in enough oxygen to fuel itself aerobically, so increases its use of glycogen, producing more lactate. After about 60–90 minutes at this intensity, the body will need additional fuel.

### Fast- and slow-twitch muscle
The two basic types of fibre that muscles are made of. Fast-twitch muscle fibres contract quickly but tire rapidly, generating short bursts of strength or speed, such as in sprinting. Slow-twitch muscle fibres contract slowly but take longer to tire, so are useful for endurance activities such as long-distance running or cycling.

### Glycogen
A form of carbohydrate stored by your body for use as fuel. The quantity you can store varies, although you can train your muscles to increase the amount they can absorb (see p.91). Running out of glycogen causes hypoglycaemia (low blood sugar), also known as "bonking" or "hitting the wall".

### Lactate
A by-product of the metabolic processes your body uses to create the fuel it needs during aerobic and anaerobic exercise. The level of lactate produced increases during higher-intensity anaerobic exercise.

### Lactate threshold
The point at which your body produces lactate faster than it can metabolize (process) it, which happens during high-intensity anaerobic exercise. The build-up of lactate in your muscles stops them taking on any more oxygen, causing them to tire. Training at, or slightly below, your lactate threshold can raise your threshold, along with your VO2 max.

### Vasodilation
The widening of your blood vessels, which enables your heart to pump additional oxygen and nutrients to your muscles during exercise, while also allowing lactate to be dispersed quickly through your bloodstream (see p.69).

### vVO2 max
Your velocity (v) at your maximal uptake of oxygen: the maximum volume (V) of oxygen (O2) that your body can process as you swim, bike, or run. The higher your vVO2 max, the better your aerobic fitness (see pp.78–79).

---

**TRAINING LEVEL**

## 1 EASY
**50–60% of HR max**
A low-intensity training level often used in long, steady distance (LSD) training. A slower pace than the race pace for all triathlon disciplines, it increases your aerobic fitness in preparation for higher intensity work.

## 2 TEMPO
**60–70% of HR max**
This level involves training at a reasonable, medium-intensity pace, as you start to find your rhythm. Level 2 is below race pace for most triathlon distances, but at or around race pace for Ironman, and sometimes for Half Ironman running too.

## 3 THRESHOLD
**70–80% of HR max**
This the main training level for high-intensity work, becoming stressful after about 6–12 minutes (compared with c.60 minutes at Tempo). Level 3 is at or around race pace for Sprint and Olympic distance, and also for Half Ironman swimming and cycling.

## 4 vVO2 MAX
**80–90% of HR max**
Training at this level an only be sustained effectively for about 6–12 minutes. In competition, it is what elite swimmers refer to as "first buoy pace". Reaching the first buoy quickly is crucial to achieving a fast race; the race pace drops to Level 3 from there onwards.

## 5 MAXIMAL
**90–100% of HR max**
This level involves working at maximum intensity, so it is extremely demanding on the body, and can only be sustained for 150–200m (165–220yd) in the water, 90 seconds on a bike, and 200–400m (220–440yd) on a run. It is too high-intensity to be used in a race.

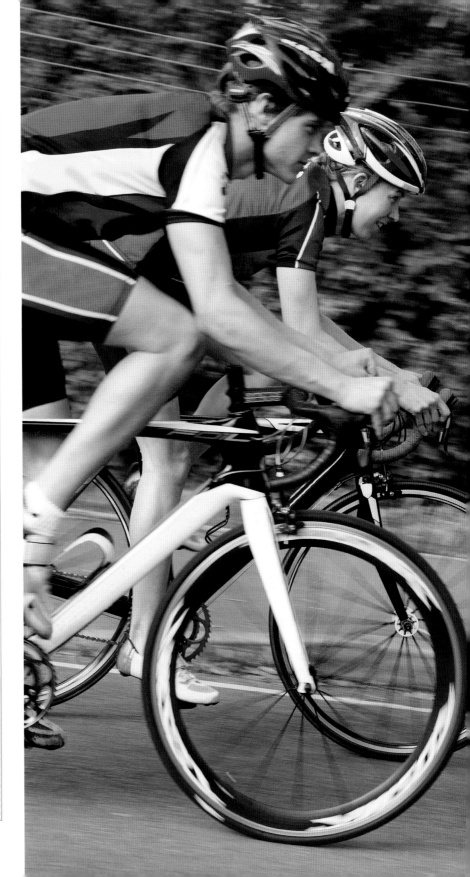

- Low-intensity aerobic exercise
- Increases your body's efficiency in carrying oxygen to your muscles
- Improves your body's ability to use its glycogen and fat stores for energy (and particularly fat over longer distances)
- Boosts your overall aerobic fitness
- Enables you to think technically
- Can be used for recovery training

- Aerobic exercise of a steady rhythm
- Develops your basic endurance levels, as it can be stressful over longer periods
- Increases your body's efficiency in delivering oxygen to your muscles
- Encourages fat-burning but your body uses more glycogen (so ensure you take on enough fuel to avoid hypoglycaemia)
- Boosts overall aerobic fitness

- Aerobic moving to anaerobic exercise
- Increases the production of lactate in your muscles, although usually still within your lactate threshold
- Develops your overall stamina
- Improves your ability to cope with the stress of working at a higher intensity
- The optimum level for adjusting to the effort, rhythm, and feel of race pace

- Intense anaerobic exercise
- Improves your body's overall energy efficiency, and your level of maximum possible performance
- The ideal intensity for increasing your vVO2 max and lactate threshold levels
- Improves your mental toughness and the overall efficiency of your training, due to the stress of the high intensity

- Very intense anaerobic exercise
- Used correctly, improves your speed, energy efficiency, strength, and level of maximum possible performance
- Increases your vVO2 max level
- Highly stressful and demanding; you should train sparingly at this level, and ensure that you rest properly afterwards

# GLOSSARY

**Acute injury** An injury that occurs suddenly, for example a ruptured Achilles tendon.

**Aero bars** Bars either added to, or integrated into, the handlebar system on a tri bike, designed to improve aerodynamics.

**Aerobic** A process that requires oxygen. It is used to describe low- to moderate-intensity exercise over an extended period of time that maintains an increased *heart rate*. Running a long distance at a moderate *pace* is an example of aerobic exercise.

**Aerobic capacity** The body's ability to take in, transport, and convert oxygen to energy during exercise. See also *VO2 max*.

**Aerodynamic** Designed to move easily though the air.

**Anaerobic** A term used to describe high-intensity exercise that demands more oxygen than the body can supply. Anaerobic literally means "without oxygen". Sprinting is an example of anaerobic exercise.

**Antagonistic muscles** A pair of muscles that work against each other to create movement. When one muscle contracts, the other relaxes. The biceps and triceps are examples of antagonistic muscles.

**Anterior** Located at the front.

**Bilateral breathing** A breathing technique in swimming that involves breathing on both sides (typically every three, five, or seven strokes).

**Biomechanics** The study of how the body functions in relation to movement.

**Brick session** A type of *training session* in which an athlete goes from one triathlon discipline straight into another (e.g. bike to run). It is used to simulate race experience and is designed to get the body used to switching sports quickly.

**Cadence** In cycling, cadence refers to pedalling speed measured in *revolutions per minute (rpm)*. It also refers to the strike rate in running and stroke rate in swimming.

**Carbohydrate** A substance found in food such as bread, potatoes, and pasta. It is used by the body as fuel to provide energy. See also *glucose*.

**Cardiovascular** Relating to the heart and blood vessels in the circulatory system.

**Chronic injury** An injury that develops over a long period, and may also be slow to heal.

**Cleat** A metal or plastic fitting that attaches to the sole of a cycling shoe and clips into the pedal. A built-in mechanism releases the foot in an accident. This pedal system is also known as "clipless".

**Cool-down** Slow or gentle stretching exercises performed after a hard *workout* or race to help the body recover. See also *flushing*.

**Core** The area of the body between the ribs and the hips and buttocks. This group of muscles supports and stabilizes the torso. See also *trunk*.

**Draft** To tuck in behind or just to the side of another runner, swimmer, or cyclist letting that person set the pace and block the wind. Drafting in the bike leg is illegal in most age group triathlons.

**Drag** Water or air resistance that reduces an athlete's speed.

**Drills** Specific and repetitive exercises that are used to improve an athlete's technique and efficiency.

**Economy of motion** A measure of how much oxygen an athlete uses at any given speed. See also *running economy*.

**Electrolytes** Essential minerals stored in the body, such as sodium, zinc, and potassium. Electrolytes are lost through sweating.

**Endurance** The ability of the muscles to work for an extended period of time without tiring.

**Endurance training** A type of low-intensity training designed to increase stamina and improve the body's *aerobic capacity*.

**Fartlek** A type of *training session* that includes periods of faster running alternated with slower running to add variety. Fartlek is a Swedish word meaning "speedplay".

**Fat-adapting** A process that involves adapting diet and training the body to use fat as fuel.

**Flexibility** The range of movement at, across, or around a joint. An athlete's flexibility can be improved by stretching.

**Flushing** A process during a *cool-down* that involves gently contracting and relaxing the muscles to help blood circulate to fatigued muscles.

**Force work** A type of *training session* that uses resistance to increase muscle strength and stamina.

**Functional threshold power (FTP)** The maximum power that an athlete can sustain during exercise over a one-hour period. Cyclists often measure FTP with a *power meter*.

**Glucose** A basic form of sugar into which all *carbohydrates* are converted in the body. Excess glucose is stored in the liver and muscles as *glycogen*.

**Glycaemic index (GI)** Ranking of *carbohydrate*-containing foods based on their overall effect on blood *glucose* levels. Foods that are absorbed slowly have a low GI rating, while foods that are more quickly absorbed have a higher rating.

**Glycogen** The form in which *glucose* is stored in the body, usually in the liver and muscles. When your glycogen levels fall during *aerobic* exercise, you will begin to feel fatigued.

**GPS (Global Positioning System)** A navigation system that uses satellites to determine the exact location and velocity of a person at any point in time. A GPS watch is used by athletes to record data such as *heart rate* and speed.

**Heart rate (HR)** The number of times the heart beats per minute.

**Heart-rate monitor** A device that records and displays the *heart rate* during exercise.

**Hill training** A type of *training session* designed to improve *strength endurance* and speed. Cycling or running up steep hills also helps to improve an athlete's *lactate threshold*.

**Hydrodynamic** Designed to move smoothly and easily through water.

**Hypoglycaemic crash** Extreme fatigue and loss of energy caused by depleted *glycogen* levels. It is commonly known as "bonking" or "hitting the wall".

**Hyponatraemia** A medical condition that occurs when there is a low concentration of sodium in the body fluids. It is usually caused by drinking excessive amounts of water without replacing *electrolytes* after prolonged physical activity.

**Interval training** A type of *training session* where periods of high-intensity exercise are interspersed with periods of lower-intensity activity. It is designed to strengthen the heart muscle so that oxygen can be pumped round the body more efficiently.

**ITU (International Triathlon Union)** The international governing body for triathlon. It was founded in April 1989 in Avignon, France, the site of the first official world championships.

**Kinetic chain** The interconnected chain of muscles, joints, tendons, ligaments, and nerves that work together to produce movement.

**Lactate** A by-product of the body's use of *glucose* by muscle cells. Its production is increased during intense exercise.

**Lactate threshold** The point during high-intensity exercise when *lactate* is produced faster than it can be removed from the bloodstream. The body can be trained to raise its lactate threshold through exercise.

**Lateral** Located on or extending towards the outer side of the body.

**Level** A measurement of the intensity and duration of a *training level*. In this book, the levels range from 1–5, with Level 5 being the most difficult.

**Lumbar** Relating to the lower part of the back.

**Maximum heart rate** The highest number of times your heart can beat in a one-minute period.

**Medial** Located on or extending towards the middle.

**Moisture wicking** Fabric designed to absorb moisture, especially sweat, from the skin's surface.

**No man's land** A particularly tough or demanding period during a race or training session. It typically occurs halfway through a discipline in a triathlon.

**Overload** A process in which additional stress is placed on the body to improve performance. Overload is designed to help an athlete adjust to training at a higher *level*.

**Over-reaching** Training beyond your limit. Over-reaching is fine in the short-term but it can lead to *overtraining* if continued for an extended period of time.

**Overtraining** A condition caused by training too much, leading to fatigue, burn-out, and/or injury.

**Pace** A measure of speed, usually described as the number of minutes taken to run a mile.

**Pick ups** Training at around race pace for a short period of time.

**Posterior** Located behind.

**Power** The ability to exert the maximum force in the shortest possible time. Power is generated by the action of the muscles.

**Power meter** An electrical gauge fixed to a bike that measures the energy output of a cyclist (usually measured in watts).

**Pre-hab** A series of exercises designed to strengthen muscles

and reduce the risk of injury during training.

**Progression** A gradual increase in workload to improve performance.

**Race pace** The speed an athlete needs to achieve and sustain in order to complete a specific race in the desired time.

**Rate of perceived exertion (RPE)** A simple method of measuring the intensity of exercise based on how hard you feel your body is working. The scale rates exercise intensity from 1 to 10, with 10 being maximum effort.

**Recovery** A period of low-intensity exercise following a hard *training session* to allow the body to recover and repair any damage.

**Rehabilitation** The process of recovering fully from injury.

**Repetitions (reps)** The number of times an athlete performs a specific exercise without stopping for a break. See also *set*.

**Resistance training** A type of training that uses resistance (such as weights, dumbbells, or resistance bands) to increase muscle strength and overall fitness.

**Rest** The suggested length of the *recovery* period between individual *sets* in a *training session*.

**Resting heart rate** The rate at which the heart beats when the body has been at rest.

**Revolutions per minute (rpm)** See *cadence*.

**Rollers** A training device consisting of rolling cylinders that enables a cyclist to ride on a bike (often indoors) without moving forwards.

**Running economy** A measure of how much oxygen an athlete uses during exercise over a given time. A greater running economy means faster speeds. See also *economy of motion*.

**Run-off** A type of workout that involves going straight from the bike (off bike) into the run. Unlike a *brick*

*session*, run-offs are completed when the legs are fatigued after a long ride. Practising run-offs trains the leg muscles to adjust to switching disciplines.

**Set** The number of *repetitions* that an athlete completes. Sets are separated by a short period of *rest*.

**Sighting** To check your position in open water by raising your head just above the surface of the water and keeping your eyes forwards.

**Specificity training** A method of training that is tailored to the specific needs of the sporting activity to achieve the best results.

**Split** The time taken to complete an individual section of a race or *workout*.

**Strength endurance** The ability to exercise with *resistance* over an extended time period. Muscular strength endurance can be improved by *strength training*.

**Strength training** A type of training that uses *resistance* through bodyweight, weights, or paddles (in water) to build muscular strength and *endurance*.

**Strike rate** In running, the number of times one foot hits the floor per minute.

**Synovial fluid** A thick liquid that lubricates a joint, enabling it to move easily.

**Tapering** Reducing the volume training prior to a race.

**Tempo runs** Running sessions performed at a *pace* that an athlete can sustain comfortably for about an hour.

**Thoracic** Relating to the chest area.

**Threshold runs** Running sessions that are performed at a higher intensity than normal to raise an athlete's *lactate threshold*. Training at lactate-threshold teaches the body to use oxygen more efficiently.

**Time trial** An individual race against the clock over a medium distance.

**Torque** The amount of force needed to make the pedals rotate on a bike.

**Training level** See *Level*.

**Training session** A period of fitness training that consists of a *warm-up*, *drills*, a main activity (the focus of the session), and a *cool-down*. The main activity usually involves swimming, cycling, or running, but can also involve strength and conditioning exercises.

**Transition area** The area where athletes change disciplines during a triathlon, and (before the race) set up equipment such as bikes, towels, water, nutrition, and running shoes.

**Trunk** The part of the body that includes the thorax (chest) and abdomen. See also *core*.

**Turbo trainer** A training device that holds the rear wheel of a bike to keep it stationary, thus allowing it to be used for indoor training.

**Underperformance syndrome** A cycle of fatigue and poor performance caused by overtraining.

**Visualization technique** A type of training technique in which you imagine the movement patterns your body will perform during a particular discipline - or your progress through the entire race.

**VO2 max** The maximum capacity of an individual's body to transport and use oxygen during exercise. VO2 max reflects the physical fitness of the individual. V-volume, O2-oxygen, max-maximum. See also *aerobic capacity*.

**vVO2 max** The velocity at which your body achieves its *VO2 max* (maximal oxygen uptake).

**Warm-up** Essential exercises that loosen the joints and muscles and prepare them for exercise. A warm-up can also include *visualization*.

**Wicking** See *moisture wicking*.

**Workout** A session of physical exercise or training. See also *training session*.

# INDEX

# ACKNOWLEDGMENTS

**ABOUT THE AUTHOR**

James Beckinsale (MSc and BTA Level 3) is one of the UK's leading high-performance triathlon coaches. Founder of Optima Racing Team in London, he has been training novice, age-group, and elite athletes in all distances, from sprint to Ironman, since 1998. His athletes have competed and achieved podium success at all levels, including European and World championships, Commonwealth Games, and Olympic Games.

**PUBLISHER'S ACKNOWLEDGMENTS**

DK would like to thank the following for their kind assistance:
**Editorial:** Claire Cross, Gareth Jones, Megan Kaye, Sabina Mangosi, Toby Mann, Andrea Mills, and Darrelle Parker; Corinne Masciocchi (proofreading); and Vanessa Bird (indexing).
**Design:** Mandy Earey and Simon Murrell.
**Hair and make-up stylist:** Alli Williams.
**Models:** Optima athletes Archie St Aubyn, Natalie Thomas, and Oliver Woods; Donna Louise, Martin Mednikarov, Christopher Pym, and Emily Rogers of Needhams Models.

All triathlon event photos were taken at the AJ Bell London Triathlon 2015.

All images © Dorling Kindersley